PRAISE FOR *ORIGINAL LIGHT*

"Snatam is a living example of an ecstatic soul, and her book is a trans-mission of love and devotion, shared with supreme totality. The beauty and purity that shines through her music is evident here, throughout the book, in her words and in her teachings. Allow her to inspire you, as she has done for so many of us and for so many years."

DEVA PREMAL
sacred chant artist

"If you've been enchanted by Snatam's transformative singing voice, you may be even more transfixed by her author's voice. She teaches here about Kundalini Yoga, but she does so through her personal experience, through stories that say much more than theories and instructions. In this book she found the right sound and the perfect inflections to move readers to discover their own spiritual meaning through traditional practices. I found this book enchanting, comfort-ing, and profoundly instructive."   **THOMAS MOORE**
author of *Care of the Soul* and *A Religion of One's Own*

"When I first sat down to read this book, I was intimidated by the devotion Snatam has to her spiritual practice. Waking up at 3:15 a.m.? Chanting and meditating for two hours? This was not something I could pull off! But within a few sentences, I knew that Snatam's embrace was so wide and wise, that we all can fit within the deep spiritual practices she offers. There is so much kindness and inspiration in this book. Snatam has done the hard work of mining ancient meditative practices and bring-ing them up to us, to use however we can, to make our lives better. She asks the question, 'Do you want to be your true self, or do you want to continue to live in a state of action and reaction?' And then she gives us ways to choose truth, positivity, light, and peace—for ourselves and our families and the world. She's a teacher for our times."

ELIZABETH LESSER
cofounder of the Omega Institute and author of *The Seeker's Guide*
and *Broken Open: How Difficult Times Can Help Us Grow*

"Back in the 60s, when I was searching for a practice and spirit-based lifestyle, this is the book I wanted. It tells the hows and the whys of these sacred techniques and is inspiring as well. It is a significant exposition of Yogi Bhajan's teachings on this subject."

NIRVAIR SINGH KHALSA
CEO of the Kundalini Research Institute, Level Three Lead Trainer in Kundalini Yoga as taught by Yogi Bhajan®, and author of *Ten Light Bodies of Consciousness* and *The Art, Science, and Application of Kundalini Yoga*

"Snatam Kaur has created a wonderful narrative about the practice of Kundalini Yoga. I am deeply touched by her commitment to her *sadhana*—spiritual practice— which shows in her voice and music that has captured many hearts and minds. My own spiritual practice of Raja Yoga confirms Snatam's views that we are in a unique time in the world, what she references as the Aquarian Age. Many are awakening to the reality that there is more to life than a materialistic consciousness. This seems to be a time of great change as humanity moves closer to experiencing God, where instruments like Snatam will gift us with a good read of a practice than can help us become better people."

SISTER JENNA
founder and director of the Brahma Kumaris Meditation Museum I & II, host of the *America Meditating Radio Show*, and recipient of the President's Lifetime National Community Service Award

"This book is precious, exquisite, and universal. The practices, chants, and recitations nourish and nurture body and soul, gently awaken us to our divine nature, and help us to evolve into the fullness of our being. The Sufis say, 'The true teacher kindles the light; the oil is already in the lamp.' Snatam Kaur is a rare genuine teacher who has devoted her life to service."

IMAM JAMAL RAHMAN
teacher and author of *Spiritual Gems of Islam*

ORIGINAL LIGHT

ORIGINAL LIGHT

the Morning Practice of
Kundalini Yoga

SNATAM KAUR

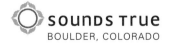

sounds true
BOULDER, COLORADO

Sounds True
Boulder, CO 80306

Music produced and published by:
Spirit Voyage Music
© and ℗ Spirit Voyage Publishing
spiritvoyagerecords.com

Published 2016

Cover design by Jennifer Miles
Book design by Beth Skelley
Illustrations © 2016 Mandy Hurwitz
Author photos: front and back covers © Eileen Escada, back flap © Jo Ann Manolis

Photo of Yogi Bhajan, courtesy of © The Teachings of Yogi Bhajan
Painting of the Naad Yogi, courtesy of Hector Jara, facebook.com/atmakundalini
Drawings of yoga postures by Mandy Hurwitz, with assistance from Sopurkh Singh Khalsa
"Long Time Sun" by Mike Heron (Warner-Tamerlane, 2004). Used by permission of Alfred Music.

Printed in Canada

Library of Congress Cataloging-in-Publication Data
Names: Snatam Kaur, 1972- author.
Title: Original light : the morning practice of kundalini yoga / Snatam Kaur.
Description: Boulder, CO : Sounds True, 2016. | Includes bibliographical references.
Identifiers: LCCN 2015034112 | ISBN 9781622035977 (hardcover)
Subjects: LCSH: Kuṇḍalinī. | Spiritual life.
Classification: LCC BL1238.56.K86 S57 2016 | DDC 294.6/436—dc23
LC record available at http://lccn.loc.gov/2015034112

Ebook ISBN 978-1-62203-636-3
Enhanced ebook ISBN 978-1-62203-719-3

10 9 8 7 6 5 4 3 2 1

This book is dedicated to my spiritual teacher, the Siri Singh Sahib,
also lovingly known as Yogi Bhajan.
Who else would have inspired such a journey?

CONTENTS

CONTENTS

INTRODUCTION

We live by the beat of the heart. When a baby cries, the mother places the baby on her chest, and the baby is comforted by her heartbeat. The mother, in turn, tunes in to this rhythm and determines what the baby needs. A steady rhythm not only comforts us, but also brings us to our own sense of inner knowing and truth. It is through a daily spiritual practice that is consistent, like the heartbeat, that we change the psyche to know—on an elemental, psychic, physical, chemical, and spiritual level—that we are in fact putting the soul first.

One name for any spiritual practice done with dedication is *Sādhanā*. I have practiced Sādhanā in one shape or form for most of my life. Now at forty-two years of age, am I an enlightened being? Well, hardly. However, I remember my spiritual teacher, Yogi Bhajan, saying, "If you want to be enlightened, be a light!" And while I can't read Auras, or read your mind, or know what will happen to me tomorrow, or even why it happened to me yesterday, I do have a light to tap into, every day. This light permeates my life and guides it, without question, with love. This light brings me tremendous joy and peace, and is without a doubt my saving grace. It gives me a way to shift my inner paradigm toward my Dharma: to live in service to all through my life, my work, and my being.

What I offer to you in these pages is my daily practice—the Aquarian Sādhanā—a householder's way to experience that original and most beautiful light every day. It takes about two and a half hours to complete, or about one-tenth of a day. I remember Yogi Bhajan saying that if we give one-tenth of our day to God, God gives Himself or Herself totally to us for the rest of the day. The Sādhanā includes a wake-up routine, a recitation, yoga, chanting, prayer, and finally a conscious act of surrendering to the Divine. There is also a component of community included that is crucial; the Sādhanā is more potent in the company of others and also supports the growth of spiritual community.

The Aquarian Sādhanā is for people of all walks of life. It is not based on religious beliefs; it is based on a yogic science of life. Where there are Sikh practices offered, we learn through the sacred tradition and the universal essence within these teachings that can nourish and heal us all. In fact, whatever your walk of life may be, I believe that this practice can enhance and support the essence of your self, of who you are and what you believe in.

The Aquarian Sādhanā was given to us by Yogi Bhajan. Born in Pakistan, he became a master of Kundalini Yoga at the age of sixteen. When he was eighteen, Yogi Bhajan and his family made the journey to Delhi after the Partition of India. After raising three children with his wife, Bibiji Inderjit Kaur, and having a successful career in the military, Yogi Bhajan was drawn to the West in 1969 to share his yogic knowledge as a way to dedicate his life to service. With Kundalini Yoga, he steered thousands of young people away from drugs by helping them achieve genuine connection and healthy daily lives.

Today, there are thousands of teachers in almost every country, sharing incredible healing experiences that Yogi Bhajan first seeded in his Kundalini Yoga classes. Although he offered this technology to people

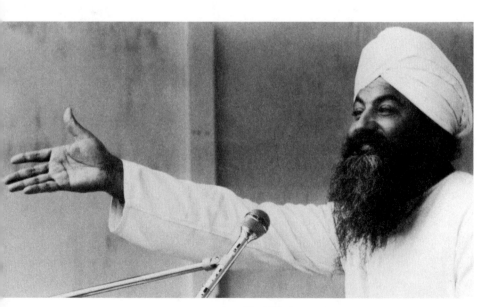

Yogi Bhajan

of all walks of life, Yogi Bhajan was a notably devoted Sikh. Many of the Mantras held within the Sikh tradition are also experienced within this Kundalini Yoga tradition. What I share with you here is specifically what I learned from my teacher Yogi Bhajan (and is referred to as Kundalini Yoga as taught by Yogi Bhajan).

He also taught the Sikh lifestlye in such a way that many became Sikhs, and an entire spiritual movement was awakened in the West. Yogi Bhajan's work was recognized by the ruling religious Sikh organization called the Shiromani Gurdwara Parbandhak Committee. In recognition and support of his service to Sikhs in the West, they gave him the title of Siri Singh Sahib. It was clear that the Universe wanted him to serve Sikhs and people of all walks of life.

My parents began to study with Yogi Bhajan right around the time I was born in 1972 (he gave me the name Snatam, which means "universal friend to all"). My mother tells me that when I was a baby, in the middle of one of Yogi Bhajan's classes, I began babbling away in a flow of excited yet unintelligible words. My mother, worried that it would disturb the class, began frantically walking with me in the back of the room, trying to quiet me down.

"You'll get your turn to teach soon!" Yogi Bhajan chided me from the stage. Everyone laughed. My mother relaxed and let me be. And so my relationship with my spiritual teacher began in this lifetime.

In 1992, Yogi Bhajan offered the Aquarian Sādhanā to help us householders thrive and remain balanced in a world with ever-increasing information, technology, and sources of stress and pressure. He knew that we would need a sense of connection and love not only within ourselves, but also within our larger communities.

HOW TO USE THIS BOOK

The intention of this book is to give you everything you need to engage in the Aquarian Sādhanā, either alone or with your family, friends, or community. In chapters 1 through 3, we explore the foundations of the practice. The idea here is to give you a working knowledge of Kundalini Yoga to empower you to understand experiences that may arise and inspire you to try out a practice, and perhaps sustain it in the long run. In chapters 4 through 8, we go into each of the five stages of the practice. In chapter 9, we look at "presence of self," something I think is possible for anyone to master. In chapter 10, we finally explore how you can do the Aquarian Sādhanā with your family and how doing so can support and nourish communities.

We have made a deliberate choice to include the Jap Ji text in appendix A so that you will have all the resources to do the Sādhanā and also enjoy the benefits of this beautiful writing. Since Jap Ji is a sacred text, I request you keep this book off of the floor as you use it, perhaps on a cushion or stand, in alignment with the traditions that hold Jap Ji in honor. To conclude this book, appendix B offers nine of my favorite Kundalini Yoga sets, appendix C provides the words for all of the chants that are in the Aquarian Sādhanā, and appendix D gives you a daily prayer called Ardās. You will also find two CDs I created with my band called *Light of the Naam with Long Ek Ong Kar* and *Jap Ji Meditation*. The first includes all of the chants for the morning practice; the second is my recitation of Jap Ji for your reference.

One way to use this book and accompanying CDs is to dive deeply into some areas right away and just soak your toes in the shallow end of other areas for a while. I suggest putting the music and recitation on in your home right away to let the positive energy begin flowing. Please take your time with this book and allow for reflection as needed.

As you begin with the stages of the practice and encounter something that would be a lifestyle change for you, I invite you to try it out and see how it feels. It is possible to experience major inner shifts by making just a few modifications to your daily life. Perhaps you could read this book with a partner or friend and try the practice out together so that when the major shifts occur, you can share your experiences with each other.

As I mentioned, there are nine different Kundalini Yoga sets offered here, all with different energies and purposes. I invite you to sit in the center of your being, feel which set draws you in on a particular day, and engage with that one. Our internal wisdom meter is actually quite accurate when we listen to it. I love these sets, and they are an active part of my week. Depending on the day, there is a good chance that I am practicing one of them.

As you read about the chants and come to understand their meanings as they apply both to your life and to your soul space, focus on those you feel most drawn to. Like water, these chants will only flow into spaces where there is an opening.

After you have gained knowledge of the practice, it's up to you to decide how to integrate it into your life. Of course, I recommend doing the whole Aquarian Sādhanā. However, even just a thirty-minute practice is a wonderful place to start. Whatever you start, I recommend you do it every day for at least forty days, as it takes this long for notable transformation to begin. If you are already practicing the Aquarian Sādhanā, perhaps this book will help you to go deeper in your experience, as it has for me in the process of writing it. You may also have no intention of integrating any of these practices into your life. That's okay, too; I also wrote this book with you in mind. We are all just travelers together in the cosmic journey called life. If nothing else, perhaps some spark of joy will come out of the story of my practice and will inspire you along the way.

PRONUNCIATION GUIDE

Throughout this book, a number of words have been transliterated from the original Gurmukhī (a sacred language developed in India in the sixteenth century) into Roman letters. Through the process of working with these words, I came to realize how important it is to try to stay true to the original written text. My goal is to preserve the original pronunciation and make it much easier to understand the root meanings by keeping to the original script.

There are numerous sounds that one could only understand by actually learning the original Gurmukhī language; I have chosen not to illustrate those sounds here with the use of Roman letters. I felt it would have created unnecessary confusion. If you have the opportunity to learn Gurmukhī, I highly recommend it for deepening your meditation experience. This sacred language offers tremendous joy and bliss.

Please use the following charts to help with your pronunciation of Gurmukhī.

Vowels

SYMBOL	CARRIER	TRANSLITERATION	EXAMPLE OF SOUND
none	ਅ	a	like the "a" in *about*
T	ਆ	ā	like the "a" in *father*
f	ਇ	i	a sound in between "i" as in *bit* and "e" as in *egg*
		e	the transliteration letter "e" may be used for this symbol at times
ੀ	ਈ	ī	like the "ee" in *beet*
_	ਉ	u	like the "u" in *put*
ੂ	ਊ	ū	like the "oo" in *soon*
ੇ	ਏ	ay	like the "ay" in *say*
ੈ	ਐ	ai	like the "a" in *hand*
ੋ	ਓ	o	like the "o" in *go*
ੌ	ਔ	au	this sound would be produced by sounding out the transliteration letter "ā" with your mouth in an *O* shape

Vowel Combinations

Vowels often appear side by side, noted here with hyphens as in "i-ā," "ā-ay," and "o-ī." Pronounce these vowels sequentially in a smooth manner.

Consonants

The consonant sounds are fairly self-explanatory as seen in this chart, although some of them do not appear in the English language. I explain some of these sounds after the chart. Please use the included Jap Jī recording to follow along with the text as a reference point.

ਸ	s	ਦ	d
ਹ	h	ਧ	dh
ਕ	k	ਨ	n
ਖ	kh	ਪ	p
ਗ	g	ਫ	ph
ਘ	gh	ਬ	b
ਙ	n(g)	ਭ	bh
ਚ	ch	ਮ	m
ਛ	chh	ਯ	y
ਜ	j	ਰ	r
ਝ	jh	ਲ	l
ਞ	ñ	ਵ	v or w
ਟ	t̲	ੜ	r̲
ਠ	t̲h	ਸ਼	sh
ਡ	d̲	ਖ਼	(kh)
ਢ	d̲h	ਗ਼	(g)
ਣ	n̲	ਜ਼	z
ਤ	t	ਫ਼	f
ਥ	th		

Retroflex Consonants

You can pronounce retroflex consonants by touching the tip of your tongue to the roof of your mouth half an inch back, toward the soft palate. These consonants are noted with an underline, for example t̲, t̲h, d̲, d̲h, n̲, and r̲.

Rolling the "R"

Roll the "r" as you would in Spanish. The sound resembles the "t" in *city*. For the retroflex "r̠," the sound is like the "rd" in the word *hard*.

Subtle Vowel Sounds

In Gurmukhī, if a word ends in a consonant, there is always a subtle sound at the end of the word, a form of rise or lilt. Please refer to the recording to hear this. In the study of Gurmukhī, one can go into much more detail with this, but I have not noted it here. In the case where the word ends with an "h" consonant, there are subtle vowel sounds that are noted as such:

(u) like the "u" in *put*
(i) like the "i" in *bit*

THE INSTRUMENT OF YOU

Yogi Bhajan taught that with every wink of an eye, there are a thousand thoughts.[1] Only one of those thoughts becomes articulated into language, and those words become action. Underneath all of those thoughts is a baseline energy, an unstruck sound, a silence named *Anahat*. In this silence we do not have to do or think anything; we can just be. It is a pure state of meditation where we open the doors to merge with God, to *be* God. We enter a flow that is beyond thoughts, ideas, and actions; the flow just is, and we can just be.

What is the vibratory frequency of that inner space? You can find out. And from that discovery, you can create such a beautiful melody that the Universe will bend its ear to listen. But you must work on the instrument, the *you*. If you play a violin made by the Stradivarius family, the most beautiful sound will come out. If you take a rinky-dink Suzuki-student violin and play it, you can only make it sound so good. That Stradivarius has been worked on. The wood is the highest quality possible. The body is shaped just so. The strings are finely made. Everything has been masterfully created so that when it is played, an amazing sound comes forth. Its Anahat, the unstruck sound, is ready to directly touch the heart.

That is exactly what spiritual practice is. You become a kind of Stradivarius violin so that when the Creator plays you, you make incredible music. The sound that comes out will be divine. Why? Your baseline, inner-core vibration has been given space to exist, and your body and mind are finely tuned to carry that vibration out into the Cosmos.

~ *Chapter One* ~

THE GIFT OF PRACTICE

ਚਰਨ ਸਰਨਿ ਗੁਰ ਏਕ ਪੈਂਡਾ ਜਾਇ ਚਲ,

charan saran gur ayk paindā jā-i chal,

If you take but one step towards the Gurū,

ਸਤਿਗੁਰ ਕੋਟਿ ਪੈਂਡਾ ਆਗੋ ਹੋਇ ਲੇਤ ਹੈ ॥

satigur kot paindā āgay ho-i layt hai.

He takes a million steps towards you.

BHAI GURDĀS JĪ, *AMRIT KĪRTAN*[1]

In the early morning hours, I opened the door to the little cabin I was staying in to walk to the group Sādhanā practice just down the road. It was just me; not a soul stirred. I was living with my sister for the summer in a sacred community nestled in a valley of the Jemez Mountains of northern New Mexico. I was in my early twenties, and I felt totally safe as the cottonwood trees sang, rustling in the wind. The cool air invited me in, and as I took a deep breath, my eyes were drawn upward to the sparkling stars in the dark blue sky. It was at that moment that I fell in love with my practice. It was God's time to say hello to me, to tell me how much He loved me, and it was my time to say hello to Him, undisturbed by the hustle and bustle of the day. From that moment on—whether in a busy city, on a tropical island, in a quiet forest, or through the window of a cozy home—I have always looked for the stars and moon before beginning my practice.

Before we take a quick look at the Aquarian Sādhanā, I want to reflect on what a blessing it is just to be able to think and speak about spiritual matters. The sages tell us that it takes 8.4 million lifetimes just to obtain birth as a human. Then, as human beings, we must cycle through our various lessons until we learn them. To have the opportunity to explore matters of spirit most likely means that we have passed through quite a bit of struggle and drama. And here we are.

THE FIVE STAGES
OF THE AQUARIAN SĀDHANĀ

So, appreciating our good fortune, let's look at what the Aquarian Sādhanā actually consists of, the effects we may experience from this practice, and what engaging our spirituality in this way means to us in this modern day and age.

Stage One: Preparing for the Aquarian Sādhanā

This stage includes steps to healthy living that prepare you for the maximum benefit of the Sādhanā. You can also apply these teachings to any other spiritual practice or path. In this stage you learn how to create a sacred space, yogic guidelines for healthy elimination, a bathing method, and how to select clothing that will support your experience.

Stage Two: Jap Jī

Jap Jī is a sacred recitation from Gurū Nānak, a fifteenth-century sage from India. These saintly words describe the soul's merger with the One. After submerging in a river and entering into a meditative state, Gurū Nānak emerged after three days to share his vision that the Divine exists within everyone. He taught others to recite Jap Jī and offered it as a personal road map to our own experience of merger with the Divine.

Stage Three: Kundalini Yoga

This stage consists of a Kundalini Yoga Kriya, or yoga set, given by Yogi Bhajan. Out of the thousands of sets that he taught, this manual offers nine that I enjoy practicing in the morning. Many of these include physical movements for vitality and health, but the sets aren't just for exercise; they open our physical and mental spaces to support the somatic home of our spirits. People of all levels of yogic experience can enjoy these sets.

Stage Four: Aquarian Sādhanā Mantras

In previous stages, we have done the work of enhancing our *Shaktī*, our power. In stage four we get to experience *Bhaktī*, bliss and ecstasy. We sing seven Mantras as the sun rises, merge, and experience freedom. In other words, we open the doors of liberation with our own voices vibrating these sacred sounds.

Stage Five: Gateway to Divinity

In this stage, we bring the practice back to the Divine, balance our energy, and remain in a place of service and humility throughout the day. I will encourage you here to tap into your own spiritual tradition. For those who are interested, I will also share with you the Sikh worship service called Gurdwārā as well as a way to connect with the Gurū if you do not have a Gurdwārā to take part in. We will then learn a song of blessing for this fifth and final stage.

WHEN DOES ALL OF THIS HAPPEN?

Here's how I schedule the Aquarian Sādhanā in my life:

- At 3:15 a.m., I wake up and go through the first stage: the Kundalini yogī's wake-up routine. When I was younger, I needed a lot less time. Please keep in mind that the timing for this stage will vary from person to person.

- By 4:00 a.m., I sit in my meditation spot and begin Jap Jī (the second stage).

- Between 4:20 and 4:30 a.m., I enter the third stage with a Kriya from the Kundalini Yoga sets.

- At 5:00 a.m., I start the chanting of the fourth stage.

- Finally, by 6:15 a.m., I begin the fifth stage with the practice of Gurdwārā: I pray, receive a sacred reading, and share in communion with my family and friends.

Right after I turned forty a couple of years ago, I slipped away to get tea before our concert's sound check. A woman seated at one of the café tables stopped me.

"Excuse me, Snatam," she said, looking up from a pile of books and papers spread all over her table. "Can I ask you a question?"

"Sure!" I responded, my eyes squinting in the August sun. I had met the woman earlier and knew that she was attending our concert.

"How do you have such a good complexion?" she asked.

"I'm a vegetarian; I wake up before the sun rises, take a cold shower, and practice yoga and meditation," I replied.

"Oh," she said, looking a little disappointed. Her eyes dropped back to her papers and books. I'm guessing she would have preferred the name of a good facial cream.

THE BENEFITS OF THE AQUARIAN SĀDHANĀ

The benefits of this practice go far beyond healthy-looking skin. Here are some other ways the Sādhanā has helped me:

- **It balances the nervous system, supports a healthy spine, and improves digestion.** I often find that when my practice is consistent, I breathe more deeply throughout the day. My digestion is good, and I feel lightness in my spine. As emotional challenges arise and my nervous system gets activated, I can stay in a strong place and do not react as strongly as I might otherwise.

- **It grounds body, mind, and soul with powerful affirmations.** I know my practice has been good when one of the Mantras, or sacred chants of the practice, arises in my mind during the day. The energy of it fills me with positivity and joy, and it seems to keep my mind from distracting thoughts of fear, worry, and doubt. I find myself more present and in my center. The Mantras work as positive affirmations to remind me that the Divine exists within and all around me. They really work!

- **It helps us tap into our original light every day and meet life's challenges better.** Life can be messy, stressful, and horrible. I go through such experiences just like everyone else. However, this practice gives me a way to rise above negative sensations, if even for just a few hours. And when I descend back down into the pain and mess again, I feel lighter and stronger. The sufferings of daily life carry less charge because I have experienced a totally different reality that is full of love, strength, and joy: my orginal light. I move through difficult times with less resistance, and situations redeem themselves accordingly. Struggles seem to shift, change, and fall away.

- **It fosters meaningful connections and sacred community.** The Sādhanā has helped me create lifelong relationships, and I have felt these deep connections even after just a few mornings of meditating together. The love that arises from this practice goes beyond words, as people come together to inspire themselves and each other.

- **It encourages stillness and thereby promotes closesness to God.** As humans, we experience desires almost constantly; desire is like the very blood flowing through our body. It's natural that we pursue these desires, but they never really let up. A lot of good comes from this pursuit (for example, life itself), but chasing our wants and needs around and around puts us in constant motion. Accordingly, we're so busy with the chase that it becomes increasingly difficult to be present to the reality of our lives and who we truly are. It's well established by now that meditation promotes mental and spiritual stillness. When we become still even for just a portion of the day, we harmonize with the Universe, and the Universe begins to deliver all the joys, riches, and blessings called forth by the inner frequency of our being. And let us take it even deeper than that: What if there were nothing whatsoever to want or need? To me, the experience of feeling that nothing is lacking is the experience of God, and it is absolutely priceless. That is my soul's longing. Any morning that I fulfill that longing is an absolute blessing.

- **It clears karma.** The yogīs tell us that there are two ways to clear our karma: through *Seva* (selfless service, which we'll talk about more in chapter 10) and through Sādhanā. Let's talk about Sādhanā here.

Perhaps a thousand lifetimes ago, I lived as a selfish little worm; I crawled all over my neighbors without any regard for their well-being. The residue of those past actions are still at work today: I am still not always considerate of others, and I feel victimized when people are rude to me. Karma stays with us until we finally learn our lessons and move on. Actually, I don't know if I ever was a worm in a past life, but I kind of feel like I was. Regardless, I was probably inconsiderate at one point or another.

Now that I'm reaching my midforties, my morning practice has become the place to let my karma burn in the fire of my practice (or *Tapas,* as the yogīs call it). On a subconscious level, the practice itself brings forth the residue, the truth, and perhaps the ugliness of my past mistakes, and it asks me to look at them honestly. Morning after morning after morning, I do the work of clearing this residue away, and I gradually become lighter. When I'm in a lighter place, I can more easily identify repeating patterns during the day, and I can therefore choose not to engage in the same patterns again. This cleansing process allows me to plant whatever seeds will bring good karma, good actions, and righteous living.

WILL THE SĀDHANĀ MAKE ME A BETTER PERSON?

It never ceases to amaze me how thoroughly and completely God humbles me.

Let's say on a particular day I experience the best Sādhanā ever! It feels so incredible. Afterward, my day just seems to flow right along, and everything works so well—I am so centered, so kind, so loving, so intelligent, so witty, so considerate, and just *so* wonderful in *so* many ways. I think to myself: *Oh, it must be because I did such a good Sādhanā. Oh yes, indeed; because I did a good Sādhanā, everything is working for me.*

Until that afternoon, of course, when I ask my daughter to do something simple (like, say, sing a song in our kids yoga class) and she says no, and I utterly lose it. I try a bunch of immature techniques that don't work at all while the other kids and moms are watching! And, well, there you have it. Back at square one, and humbled again.

In fact, the more I practice, the more these types of humbling experiences seem to arise. But why? The yogīs have a saying: "The higher you climb, the farther you fall." In our practice we climb higher and higher, expanding more and more into universal consciousness, but we must not forget where we have come from. We still have to live with our feet firmly planted in the place where we started: in the elemental self where our original light comes from. God keeps checking in to see if we can manage that, and He regularly pokes us with our own brand of irritating, ego-blasting, and humiliating experiences until we firmly ground ourselves in our inner truth. The Sādhanā itself in fact brings forth areas in our psyche that need work, and we will be called to more quickly address them than otherwise through situations and circumstances that we attract.

So, to answer the question above, yes, you will become a better person. But practicing the Sādhanā will get you there by unexpected, frustrating, and delightful paths.

ਕਰਮੀ ਆਪੋ ਆਪਣੀ ਕੇ ਨੇੜੈ ਕੇ ਦੂਰਿ ॥

karamī āpo āpaṇī kay nayṛai kay dūr.

*According to their own actions, some are drawn closer,
and some are driven farther away.*

GURŪ NĀNAK, *SALOK OF JAP JĪ*

17

Our actions determine our character and therefore determine our relationship with the Divine. Our choices make all the difference. At some point, it really comes down to choice. Do you want to be your true self, or do you want to continue to live in a state of action and reaction? Can you choose to take responsibility for your own mind, for your own thoughts? Every single thought takes away from or contributes to your sense of well-being. That is why the Aquarian Sādhanā infuses our thoughts with powerful affirmations through Mantra and helps us with the glorious effects of deep breathing. We do not confront the mind; we do not control the mind; we simply infuse and saturate our mind with the original light of the self and then make the choices, moment by moment, that bring us in union with our higher consciousness.

"Now an average person has over ten trillion cells. All those cells and the projection of those cells should change and renew every 72 hours. So you are constantly renewed and given new energy to make choices. If you lied yesterday, and you lied today, but you don't lie tomorrow, you will be all right."

YOGI BHAJAN[3]

Here is one of my favorite songs that Yogi Bhajan gave to the children. It's called "I Am Happy, I Am Good," and it illustrates what I'm talking about here. Songs like this fill us with positive energy and help us make the choices we know are best for us. Please sing along! It's on our album *Feeling Good Today.*

I am happy, I am good

satinām satinām satinām jī

wāhegurū wāhegurū wāhegurū jī

Truth is God's Name within my soul and the Cosmic Soul

*Great is the experience of going from darkness (gu)
to light (rū) within my soul and the Cosmic Soul*[4]

THE AQUARIAN SĀDHANĀ
IN THE AQUARIAN AGE

Have you noticed that things seem to be moving faster and faster and it takes a certain kind of mental flexibility to keep up? Have you noticed an inherent awareness within yourself that knows the truth? Have you sensed that you don't really operate as an isolated individual, that your actions are interconnected with everyone? The yogīs tell us that we're experiencing all this because we are now in the Aquarian Age. As you might guess by its name, the Aquarian Sādhanā was developed specifically for this time period. So let's take a closer look at what the Aquarian Age means and how the Sādhanā can help us in these times.

The Aquarian Age began November 11, 1991. However, there was a transition period (a cusp period) immediately following the previous time period (the Piscean Age), and this cusp completed after two decades on November 11, 2011. So we're now officially in the Aquarian Age.

In the Piscean Age, everyone lived in a more selfish manner, really as if they were isolated individuals. We focused more on our career, making a name for ourselves, and pursuing security and power. To be frank, in the Piscean Age, we could get away with a lot more in terms of crimes against humanity and the earth. How things *looked* and *seemed* were a lot more important than how they actually *were*, so people wore a lot of masks—it was easier to wear one face on the outside but actually live in a totally different manner on the inside. It's true that people sought out spiritual teachings in the Piscean Age, but the knowledge came from faraway places like the Himalayas or the Amazon, and that knowledge was guarded closely, delivered only from master to student, or kept hidden from the world altogether.

By contrast, in the Aquarian Age we are all becoming more aware of our interconnection. Knowledge of every kind is available and easy to access. People can't just hide behind their personas any longer; either the persona is too transparent, or people are just getting tired of wearing masks and trying to connect with disguises on. It just doesn't work! And we can't dump pollutants in unknown places anymore because there are no more unknown places. So, in several ways, the Aquarian Age makes it obvious that our interior space relates very directly to our exterior space. We are not isolated any longer. Our actions affect not only us but also the vast network of human beings and environments around the world. The Aquarian Age calls us to develop spiritual stamina, clarity of character, the capacity to forgive, the ability to process our emotions, and the will to surrender to do so. We must continue to grow and change through life because it demands it of us; we need flexibility both mentally and physically.[5]

If we try to operate from the motivations and energies of the Piscean Age, it can lead to insanity in the Aquarian Age. Yogi Bhajan foresaw this, and he prepared us by offering the Aquarian Sādhanā in 1992. With this practice, we have the capacity to transform and meet the pressure of this time and space through our own inner wisdom. Yogi Bhajan would often remind us that a diamond is made simply when a lump of coal undergoes tremendous pressure. Likewise, instead of resisting the pressure of our ever-changing lives, through spiritual practice we can meet that pressure with the light of the soul. Through Tapas—the fire of our discipline—we become the shining diamond within our being. This is the promise of every soul.

We do not need to be perfect; instead, let us surrender. We do not need information, or even knowledge; instead, let us experience our own well of wisdom within. We do not need to be right; only let us be intuitive, seeing the Divine play of the One.

In ancient times, when people did not have access to computers or books, wisdom was passed down through the ages in short phrases in such a way that people could memorize them. In India, this wisdom came in the form of *Sutras*. Sutras remain powerful teaching tools today, and below are five, given to us by Yogi Bhajan for the Aquarian Age.[6] Contemplate them in your own life and explore how they might assist you.

FIVE SUTRAS FOR THE AQUARIAN AGE

1. Recognize that the other person is you.

2. There is a way through every block.

3. When the time is on you, start, and the pressure will be off.

4. Understand through compassion or you will misunderstand the times.

5. Vibrate the Cosmos; the Cosmos shall clear the path.

When you do your practice, I encourage you to write down these Sutras and place them on your external altar or on the altar of your heart. Each has at one point helped me move through the intensity of this age with ease and flow.

~ *Chapter Two* ~

SACRED SOUND AS TEACHER

ਘਟਿ ਘਟਿ ਵਾਜਹਿ ਨਾਦ ॥

ghaṭ ghaṭ vājah(i) nād.

The Sound Current of the Naad vibrates in each and every heart.

GURŪ NĀNAK, *TWENTY-NINTH PAURĪ OF JAP JĪ*[1]

In this chapter I'll explain the basic elements of sound in the Kundalini Yoga tradition.[2] In the practice of the Aquarian Sādhanā, these sound elements (specifically, Mantras) play an important role in our transformation. The practice of Mantras, or sacred chants, are pretty well known now in the West; the word *Mantra* means projection *(tra)* of the mind *(man)*. With Mantra, we project the mind into a state of infinity. Instead of stopping our mind from thinking, we meet the intensity of our thought patterns with an equal force with the Mantra. Doing so, we are then able to change the flow of our thoughts, just as a pebble creates waves in a pond. As we engage in our practice and drop the Mantra into our minds, the wave of it ripples from its origin through us. Essentially, Mantras work as positive affirmations that align the frequency of our mind and every cell, particle, and atom of our body with the original light within. When you feel it in your toes (even the funny-looking ones), when you see it in the mirror (even if your face doesn't resemble that of a magazine model's), when it vibrates through every weakness to a place of victory, and when you accept and love it whole-heartedly, *then* you have experienced Mantra.

Many of the Mantras in Kundalini Yoga are from the Gurmukhī writings of the Sikhs, but there are also Mantras in English and other languages that are from other spiritual traditions. Yogi Bhajan never really saw the practice of chanting as religious. He once said, "There are tons of Mantras—I only use those which I know will be very elementary and will work."

NAAD: SACRED SOUND CURRENT

Naad is the yogic term for the sacred sound current. It is a flow that emanates from us when we chant from our heart and spirit. *Na* means no, something with a limit, finite; *aad* means the infinite. So *Naad* is the experience of the infinite existing within the finite form. The Mantras we chant have been given to us through the experience of complete union with the One. That incredible being who recited the Mantra originally did it within a state of bliss in the physical human body, and the Mantra works for us as a road map to attain that same state in our own body, through chanting.

SHABAD GURŪ: SACRED SOUND AS TEACHER

I received an email a few years back from a woman whose husband had fought in Iraq. He experienced the horrors of war known too well by veterans all across the United States and the world. When he came back from Iraq, this soldier was clearly traumatized, but he couldn't cry—he didn't cry at all for several years. But then his wife came across our music and played a track called "Ra Ma Da Sa" one day. As the sacred sounds entered his mind and body, the man suddenly began to cry, and this long-awaited weeping began a deep healing process. So his wife wrote to thank me, particularly for my voice. I responded with gratitude that our music could help her husband in some way, but it wasn't me. The Mantra offers something much deeper than my voice, much deeper than the music.

The essence of the healing I believe her husband experienced comes from what is called "Shabad Gurū." *Sha* means ego, and *bad* means without. Gurū means that which takes us from darkness *(gu)* to light *(rū)*. Accordingly, Shabad Gurū is a sound current that comes through us when we surrender our ego, and this current brings us from darkness into light, from despair into joy, from hatred into love, from separation into union. It is the spark of change we all long for.

So that you may understand how Shabad Gurū manifested on this planet as a technology of transformation, I want to share a little bit about Sikh history with you.[3] Sikhs follow the guidance of ten Gurūs who lived in physical form. The first was Gurū Nānak. He traveled with his disciple and companion, Mardana, who played a stringed instrument called a *rabab* for Gurū Nānak while he sang his teachings. Gurū and disciple traversed the entire country of India and went as far as China, Persia, and Mecca—all on foot! Even after spending mere days with Gurū Nānak, people became transformed and felt inspired to carry on his teachings for generations to follow. Gurū Nānak's poems are beautiful, with incredible rhythm, rhyme, and deep meaning. Even if you do not understand the meaning when you hear them, the poems weave their way into your heart. Gurū Nānak taught people his songs, and the songs would remain in their heart even when he left to go to the next village. This was the birth of Shabad Gurū. Through his songs, people maintained an uplifted consciousness even without Gurū Nānak's physical presence.

This tradition continued with the second, third, fourth, and fifth Gurūs. Gurū Arjan, the fifth Gurū, compiled the writings of all five Gurūs together. In addition, Gurū Arjan included the sacred writings of Sufi, Hindu, and Muslim saints of his time into a text he called the Ādī Granth. The Ādī Granth became the physical channel for Shabad Gurū to manifest on this planet. His message was clear: the Shabad Gurū is an energy for all faiths. It was not intended to be about religion, but about pure consciousness.

After Gurū Arjan completed his work, he showed tremendous respect to the Ādī Granth. He treated it as a living and breathing entity, going so far as sleeping on the floor and giving his bed to the text. Doing so, Gurū Arjan seeded the awareness that this sacred text is a living Gurū.

Later on, when the tenth Gurū prepared to leave his body, he appointed the Gurūship to this body of writings we now call the Sirī Gurū Granth Sāhib. The Sirī Gurū Granth Sāhib is our eleventh Gurū and acts as the focal point of every Gurdwārā, or Sikh place of worship. Sikhs give the Sirī Gurū Granth Sāhib a special place in their homes.

I personally look to the Sirī Gurū Granth Sāhib for guidance, comfort, security, and joy. I often take a *Hukam*—a sacred reading—whenever I have a question that needs resolution or whenever I just need to feel a sense of connection and grace. It works for me without fail. I always receive a clear message for the exact emotions and energy that I am experiencing.

The Sirī Gurū Granth Sāhib is written in Gurmukhī, a language fashioned by Gurū Angad, the second Sikh Gurū. Gurū Angad intended that Gurmukhī function to bring healing, consciousness, awareness, and inner light. I started learning it at the age of six, when my mother taped the Gurmukhī alphabet to the backseat of our car so that I could practice on the way to school. Even today, I still consider myself a student of Gurmukhī, learning and improving my skills. And as I deepen my awareness of its nuances, Gurmukhī becomes more and more powerful for me as a meditation tool.

Many of the Mantras in the Kundalini Yoga tradition come from the Sirī Gurū Granth Sāhib, and a number of the Mantras and songs that I have recorded throughout the years come from it, as well. In this context, the term Shabad can refer to a sacred poem put to music.

Often people who listen to my albums do not understand a single word I sing, but they nevertheless feel a deep connection. This connection is the vibration of Shabad Gurū coming through.

HOW MY RELATIONSHIP
WITH SHABAD GURŪ BEGAN

When I was eighteen, Yogi Bhajan asked me to move to Los Angeles. Living just a few blocks away from his home and the community Gurdwārā, I was quite busy with work, community activities, and taking part in Yogi Bhajan's classes. Within just a few months, he gave me three essential teachings about Shabad Gurū: First, we must listen in order to truly understand ourselves, our surroundings, and the truth. Second, we must surrender our egos and allow ourselves to become channels so that the timeless wisdom of sound can come through. Third, let us sing the words of the Shabad Gurū with intention and love. Doing so saturates our being with positive vibrations so that the sum total of who we are aligns with our highest self and the Divine.

Listen

After a Gurdwārā service one Sunday afternoon, Yogi Bhajan called me to sit beside him as we all partook of the community meal. Everyone sat in rows, in the traditional way that food is served in Gurdwārā, while the servers came around with big pots of yogurt, rice, dahl, and whatever else had been prepared. The little hall was packed with at least eighty people, so there was a lot of talking and laughing going on.

I had been feeling frustrated. As an eighteen-year-old, I wanted so much to begin my life and to do something important. I wasn't clear on what I wanted to do, and I also didn't feel understood by anyone. The thoughts of frustration welled up within me, and I wished to speak to Yogi Bhajan about it. As I sat down trying to formulate my question, all of my thoughts seemed to scatter in the intensity of his presence. I couldn't even say hello; I just sat down. The servers brought all of us dahl and rice, and we began eating as I struggled to formulate my question in my mind. How could I ask him my question if I didn't even know what was going on inside me? Thought after thought ravaged me, and my frustration continued to grow. After a few moments of eating in silence, Yogi Bhajan said to me, without even looking, "Listen, listen to all of them talking."

So I did; I listened.

I began hearing the conversations around me. A man just a few feet away was talking about a movie he had recently seen. Another woman spoke of seeing some beautiful flowers on her morning walk and how she would love to grow some roses in her garden. A child cried. Someone laughed at a joke.

"Their voices flow out, like rivers, telling the story of their lives," he said, leaning over slightly so that I could hear him.

And then I truly listened without getting caught up in the details of individual conversations.

Their voices began to merge into one flow, like little ripples in a river. Talking, chattering, flowing. My heart skipped a beat as I realized the sound was life itself: their lives, pouring out, moment by moment, carrying the story of each soul. The specifics didn't matter—the sound streamed forth, guiding each soul forward into its next experience. And there I was, listening to it all with my teacher.

As I listened, my earlier frustration of not being heard and not knowing what to do with my life melted. I began to understand that it did not matter who listened to me or if anyone truly understood me. God was listening to me, as my teacher revealed when he showed me how to truly listen. What mattered was the vibratory frequency within my being, the thoughts that followed that vibration, my words, and my songs. Because then, my soul would follow, my life would follow, and all things would manifest from the vibratory frequency that I chose to produce.

Be a Channel

A few months later, Yogi Bhajan asked me and two other musicians to play music in the Gurdwārā every night. We would sing sacred songs and read the evening prayers, and someone would bring treats for everyone to share. At first, lots of people came and really seemed to enjoy themselves. Personally, I loved playing with the other musicians and hearing people's voices. It was wonderful.

However, as the weeks passed, one of the musicians got busy with work and couldn't make it any longer. We kept going, but in a couple of weeks, the *Sangat* (or sacred community) diminished from twenty to fifteen. Then, the other musician dropped out, and only ten people showed up.

I remember trying to focus on chanting a Shabad, but my eyes kept looking to the door, wondering if others would arrive. The *Sevadaars*, those who perform service at the Gurdwārā, had flung the doors open wide to the busy streets of Los Angeles. Every now and then, fire engines rolled by with their sirens drowning out our chanting. An old woman peered in, curious about our white clothing, our chanting, and then went on her way. Cars honked. Kids rode by on bikes.

As the weeks passed, fewer and fewer people attended the Gurdwārā, dwindling down at last until one evening I found myself alone with just the sound man (and I felt grateful that he at least showed up). It turns out the sound man was partially deaf—he kept turning up the sound quite a bit—and so my singing blasted out into the noisy street, as if protesting that, despite the low attendance, something truly important was happening in here! Oh, how I wanted people to come in!

But they didn't. Night after night, I kept looking to the door and hoping, but no one came. And although I vaguely noticed the Sirī Gurū Granth Sāhib sitting next to me, so beautifully decorated, along with the marble floors, flowers, exquisite pictures, and the setting sun, I was not present to any of the wonderful sights around me or even the Shabad that I was singing. I kept looking at the door. The frustration mounted as my thoughts wouldn't let up: *What is the use of this? Who am I singing for? Who am I helping? No one! Night after night, and no one is coming. I will keep singing though. My teacher asked me to, so this is what I should do* . . .

But my heart wasn't in it.

At some point, something shifted in me. To this day, I cannot describe how it happened; it was as simple as someone flipping a light switch. I suddenly remembered the teaching about listening that Yogi Bhajan gave me a few months earlier.

I listened to my thoughts; I listened to my being. I listened to the air around me, tumbling in lazy circles with the night breeze coming through the doorway. I listened to the whir of cars outside on the busy city street. All the sounds, including those within me, merged into a flowing river. I was no longer attached to the sound but became an observer, and from this place I settled to a still point within.

That is when I realized who I was and where I was. I could feel my life unfolding before me, with the sound emanating from me leading the way. At that time, the sum of my sound totalled up to frustration. It all seemed kind of comical at that moment because here I was, singing the blessed Shabad in this incredible Gurdwārā, built by my teacher and totally blessed with his presence and the presence of all those who meditated there day and night, and in the middle of it all, I was busy generating more and more frustrating thoughts. That was becoming my communication with the Universe, my ultimate request. The vibration of frustration would lead the way in the unfolding of my life unless I could produce something different.

At that moment, I made a resolution to create something positive in the beautiful space that surrounded me and in my life itself. My eyes focused on a picture on the wall: a painting of our fourth Gurū, Gurū Rām Dās. His hands pressed together in prayer at his chest, his eyes opened with a twinkle of compassion. I heard a quiet voice in my head:

"So, no one comes to see you? No one comes to see me either. Look at my wonderful colors! Look at my beautiful frame! Be here, be here like me. Be still. Be all right with no one coming to see you. You are not here for them anyway; you are here for the Gurū. That is why I am here. Be empty and hold something marvelous like the wooden frame of this picture."

I chuckled to myself. Was I going crazy? I gazed at the wooden frame painted in gold and tried it out. There was nothing else for me to do anyway. My frustrating thoughts were unbearable. So I listened to the picture's advice and became still. I stopped looking at the door, and then I sang.

And oh, what joy came through me as I sang, to God and to Gurū! I didn't need anyone else; I didn't need their approval or their presence. After all, I wasn't singing for them anyway. I felt the Gurū deeply listening to me, as He always had been, right there with me.

And it was on that day that I first understood the second act of consciousness needed when carrying the Shabad Gurū, which is to not have ego, to be a channel, a true channel of the Divine. What is a channel anyway? It's like a hose, just some simple rubber that allows something else to pass through. But the rubber hose itself is inanimate, dead. "Dead in life," as the yogīs say. It's from this place that true wisdom springs forth and from this place only that recordings are made that help a scarred veteran to cry at last.

Sing

I began to sing the Shabad now in a state of joy and love. From this place, the words began to weave in and out of my being as a dance and celebration.

As Yogi Bhajan taught us, our tongues vibrate at the roof of the mouth when we chant the Shabad Gurū. This vibration stimulates eighty-four meridian points on the roof of the mouth that send messages to our hypothalamus, an area in the brain that relates to our nervous and glandular systems.[4] Like Morse code, the rhythm of the Shabad makes a pattern in the hypothalamus that recreates the same deep meditative experience on a physical level that the Gurūs themselves experienced.

As I chanted on that beautiful evening in Los Angeles, a warmth began to grow at my heart center. A feeling of exhaltation sprang forth. I could sing forever! There was an energy within me, beyond me, above me, and all around me that had come alive. From that moment on, I knew that the Shabad Gurū was real and could manifest on this planet, that it could manifest through me or anyone willing to take the journey.

As you yourself delve into the Aquarian Sādhanā and experience the Mantras, the Naad, and the Shabad Gurū, you may also experience shifts in your conciousness. These transformations will occur exactly when you need them, and I suggest opening up to this energy with all of your heart. It may feel intimidating at first because it is always more comfortable to stay with what we know, to keep within the confines of our status quo. Try something different. I promise that you'll find something within the sacred sound that will bring you genuine transformation and become an incredible teacher in this life.

~ Chapter Three ~

A JOURNEY INTO KUNDALINI

ਰੇ ਮਨ ਇਹ ਬਿਧਿ ਜੋਗੁ ਕਮਾਓ ॥

ray man eh bidh jog kamā-o.

Oh my mind, practice yoga in this way.

ਸਿੰਙੀ ਸਾਚ ਅਕਪਟ ਕੰਠਲਾ ਧਿਆਨ ਬਿਭੂਤ ਚੜਾਓ ॥੧॥ਰਹਾਉ॥

sin(g)ī sāch akapaṯ kanṯhalā dhi-ān bibhūth charā-o. || 1|| rahā-u ||

Make truth your horn, sincerity your necklace,
and apply meditation as ashes on your body.

GURŪ GOBIND SINGH, *AMRIT KĪRTAN*[1]

Although Kundalini Yoga is very simple, it has been known to foster major life changes in people who practice it. There are three reasons for that. First, Kundalini works directly with the *Chakra* system, the energy centers along the spinal column where we can experience incredible healing, strength, and expansion. Second, we can actually experience Kundalini rising within the temple of our physical body. Third, Kundalini Yoga works on all ten of our bodies (the physical body being only one of these).

I first experienced Kundalini Yoga as a child, hissing like a snake in cobra pose. In our *ashram,* or sacred community home, we had a children's yoga class. I loved roaring like a lion and shaping my hands like lion's claws and slashing the air. Jumping like a frog was amazing fun, too—starting out squatting then hopping up and down while crying "ribbit" with each jump. After creating entire adventures in the jungle, or wherever our journey would take us that day, we would meditate; all the children sat up straight, serene, and quiet. Then we would chant with absolute inner peace, the kind that seems to last the longest when parents aren't watching. After we finished class, we felt free, happy, and joyful—there was clarity and lightness in the air. We loved to wrestle into a giggling, squealing pile. The saints and sages of the Kundalini Yoga tradition must have been pleased—the sweet Kundalini energy had clearly come through.

Kundalini means Lock of the Beloved. In my experience, the energy of Kundalini is actually very sweet, gentle, and joyful, just like the curl in a child's hair. This form of yoga includes active movements, stationary meditations, breath work, silence, chanting, and relaxation. All of this enlivens the Kundalini energy that sits at the base of the spine. When stimulated, this energy climbs the spine and leads to incredible health benefits, as well as opening us to the Divine.

This form of yoga has been traditionally taught from master to student to only a select few. Yogi Bhajan dedicated himself in service to Gurū Rām Dās, the fourth Gurū of the Sikhs, and looked to him as his direct link in the Golden Chain, a lineage carrying these sacred teachings throughout the ages.

ਰਾਜੁ ਜੋਗੁ ਤਖਤੁ ਦੀਅਨੁ ਗੁਰ ਰਾਮਦਾਸ ॥

rāj jog takhat di-an gur rām dās.

Gurū Rām Dās was blessed with the Throne of Rāj Yoga.

THE POET BATT NAL, *SIRĪ GURU GRANTH SĀHIB JĪ*[2]

Through his service to Gurū Rām Dās, Yogi Bhajan realized that Kundalini Yoga could bring joy, health, security, comfort, and peace to everyone from all walks of life, cultures, and economic classes. With great compassion, Yogi Bhajan spread these teachings all around the world, no matter where he was. On his trips, he would offer meditation instructions to flight attendants and to cab drivers when he took taxis across various cities. Not everyone was pleased that Yogi Bhajan spread these teachings so freely: some traditional practitioners even predicted that Yogi Bhajan's life would be cut short as a consequence. However, the date predicted came and went, and it became clear that the Kundalini teachings were meant to be shared with the greater public.

In Kundalini Yoga, there are an incredible number of sets, or Kriyas, for aiding with digestion, increasing brain clarity, relieving PMS, healing insomnia, and releasing depression and trauma. A Kriya is a sequence of postures and yoga techniques used to produce a particular impact on the physical body, psyche, and self. There are also teachings for consciously communicating with our families, coworkers, and fellow community members. There are Kriyas specifically for women, men, relationships, family life, pregnancy, children, and much more. There are guidelines to follow, however, so please meet with a professionally trained Kundalini Yoga therapist and stay in consultation with your doctor if you have a chronic or acute illness.

Kundalini Yoga systematically works with the basic infrastructure of any given organ system and its origins in the energy body, the Chakras. Let's take a look at the Chakra system to know how this energy can help us.

THE CHAKRA SYSTEM

When I was a teenager, Yogi Bhajan asked me to come on a teaching tour with him. We were touring through the UK, and along with about ten other people we formed a musical group (or *Jatha*) to support him. Yogi Bhajan would teach, then we would sing. The Jatha and Yogi Bhajan's entourage all rode on a huge tour bus together, and we traveled from city to city, stopping mostly at Punjabi Sikh Gurdwārās, Sikh places of worship. Thousands of Punjabi Sikhs live in the UK, as families have immigrated from India over the past two hundred years. These Gurdwārās have become important places of community and culture for Punjabi Sikhs and others.

In one such Gurdwārā, I happened to be sitting behind Yogi Bhajan about three feet back. He sat perfectly straight, with a yogī's strength of decades of practice. After he spoke and his microphone had been removed, everyone in the whole Gurdwārā joined in reciting a sacred song together. Yogi Bhajan accompanied us in chanting, and although his back faced me and his mouth was in the opposite direction, I felt the sound emanating from his spine. It was as if his whole spine was vibrating. The sound moved through me in a clear blue wave of power. It traveled in all directions, beginning from the central cord of his spine. How was this possible? We will begin to explore that question here.

The human body is an instrument of the Divine. The yogīs have identified seventy-two strings (called *Naadīs*) throughout our body that vibrate positive life force. These energy channels gather in wheel-shaped nodes (Chakras) along the spine in seven places, including an

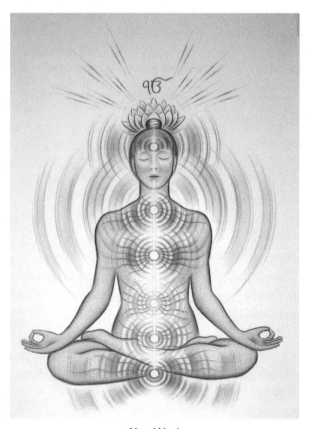

Naad Yogi

eighth location that encompasses the magnetic field that extends three to nine feet from our being. The more positive the life force that flows through us, the more empowered our Chakras are. Sometimes the Chakras are weaker in some places than others, and remedying this imbalance may require lifestyle changes. The act of engaging in a regular meditative practice like the Aquarian Sādhanā supports the Chakra system by bringing balance and nourishment to each center.[3]

First Chakra

The first Chakra sits at the end of the spine between the anus and genitals. The element of this Chakra is earth. This location determines our capacity to live in a state of self-acceptance and security; in an imbalanced state, we are plagued by insecurity and fear. When this happens, we don't feel like we belong on the earth. We may also have a hard time with our capacity to eliminate, or defecate, regularly. However, in a balanced state, we can eliminate properly and feel grounded and in touch with our elemental self. We accept ourselves, and feel secure, loyal, and stable.

Second Chakra

This Chakra resides at the sexual organs. Its element is water. This Chakra rules our capacity for creativity, and in an imbalanced state, we do not have a healthy relationship with sex. We either crave or deny it too much; perhaps we have experienced some sort of sexual trauma that has not been healed and therefore is causing a block at this location. In a balanced state, we can access the creative energy of the Universe, see the flow from the Cosmos, and know how to integrate these into our lives. Spiritual practices open us to this creative flow and foster a healthy relationship with our sexuality, whether we choose to be sexually active or not.

Third Chakra

The third Chakra sits at our navel, about an inch and a half below our belly button. The element of this Chakra is fire, and in an imbalanced state, we become greedy and full of desire. We take what isn't ours without concern for others. Or possibly our imbalance takes a different form—we don't possess enough energy to stand up for ourselves, to be ourselves. However, in a balanced state, we can digest not only our food, but also life in such a way that we take in information, process it, and locate our self in truth. Also, we have the courage to stand up for truth, stick up for ourselves, and protect others. This area is our center for personal power and commitment, so a daily spiritual practice is key to a strong and balanced third Chakra.

The yogīs teach that the longest and most arduous journey of this life is from the third Chakra to the fourth. They call it moving from the "lower triangle" to the "higher triangle." Most of humanity is stuck energetically with an imbalance in the lower triangle. Without totally balancing the first three Chakras, we cannot move into an empowered state in the higher Chakra centers.

Fourth Chakra

This is our heart center: the point of the chest level with the nipples. Its element is air. This Chakra rules our capacity to exist in a state of universal love. With a weak fourth Chakra, we may experience grief, attachment, and a desire for approval from others. In a balanced or strengthened state, we experience compassion, kindness, forgiveness, and the capacity to exist as *we* instead of just *me*. This center is our baseline energy, our Anahat: the unstruck sound from which our existence streams forth. With spiritual practice in the morning, we can open the door, thereby experiencing an open heart throughout the day.

Fifth Chakra

This Chakra resides at the throat center. Its element is ether. When our fifth Chakra comes alive, we have the capacity to communicate our truth, but when this center is weak, we become shy, suffer from voice problems, and obsess about other people's judgments. We can strengthen this Chakra by chanting sacred Mantra; these divine sound currents awaken within us the capacity to communicate with the Divine. Chanting resembles a loving language to God. The more we chant to God, the more we realize God is everywhere, and we feel that incredible truth unfolding in our lives. In this way, we begin to trust our inner knowing, and we allow our communication to come forth from this place.

Sixth Chakra

The sixth Chakra is at the Third Eye, the point between our eyebrows. When we gaze at the Third Eye, we stimulate the pituitary gland, which sits at the center of the skull, where the optic nerves cross over behind the bridge of the nose. When we practice our Sādhanā every day, we tune in to our Third Eye and can feel and see things before they happen; in this way, we free ourselves from living in the cycle of action and reaction. We find God in every moment and may even see Him wink at us here and there as life unfolds. When you live in this way, life becomes fun as little clues and hints show you that God in fact takes care of everyone, everywhere, all the time.

Seventh Chakra

This Chakra sits at the top of the head. Also known as the Crown Chakra or the Tenth Gate, when this Chakra imbalances, we feel separate from God and experience a profound fear of death. The yogīs say that this Chakra acts as our umbilical cord to God, and when it becomes activated, we can experience the energy of God directly. This is the experience of our soul in its most pure form.

Eighth Chakra

This is our Aura, the energy field around us. When all seven Chakras are strong and we enjoy a committed daily practice, our Aura radiates beautifully. The Aura acts as our first line of defense. As we move about our day, we intermingle with the Auras of all others we come in contact with. If someone feels a little off emotionally or physically, it appears first in their Aura, and their Aura affects us. If we have a strong Aura, our energy field can actually neutralize negative Auras and contribute to the healing of the other person. If our Aura is weak, however, we may take on some of that detrimental energy and become burdened by it. Through a strong practice, we can cleanse and purify our Auras, and in this way we develop a healing presence.

KUNDALINI RISING

The experience of the Kundalini energy rising feels extremely sweet. I experience it as feeling light, uplifted, clear, and content. Before the energy rises, there is a mixing of energy that brings about a state of neutrality. Through the patterns of breath created by the yoga practice and the vibration of Shabad Gurū—the sacred sound that exists within the Mantras and songs of the Kundalini Yoga tradition—the energy rises to our higher Chakra centers, and we become blessed spiritually and physically.

The process of Kundalini energy rising occurs when *Prāna* and *Apāna* unite at the navel. Prāna is the life force that moves upward, and it relates to the sun's energy, courage, and life itself. Apāna is the energy of elimination that moves downward, and it is associated with the moon's energy, receptivity, and also death. When Prāna and Apāna mix at the navel center to become neutral, the force of that interaction awakens the Kundalini energy; this is often illustrated as an awakening serpent.[4] To find your navel center, you can put your pointer finger, middle finger, and ring finger together pointing straight. Place these three fingers against your stomach with the pointer finger just below the belly button. For many of us this will be about an inch and a half below the belly button. Where the width of these three fingers end at the ring finger is an important spot. Between that spot and your lower spine rests inside your body the navel center, an etheric energy center that is in the shape of a bird's egg.[5]

Naad Yogi

40

There are probably techniques from other traditions that can make Kundalini rise, but what I am familiar with comes from the science of Kundalini Yoga as taught by Yogi Bhajan. And every morning I practice the Aquarian Sādhanā, the experience of Kundalini rising is possible. When it happens, the Kundalini rises up through the Shushmana channel and enlivens and strengthens each Chakra in my body, and this allows me to live a spiritually enriched life of service and consciousness on this planet.

When we chant the words of the Shabad Gurū in conjunction with the energy of the Kundalini energy rising, we send messages to the hypothalamus. This is an area in the brain that acts as an intermediary between the nervous system and the glandular system. It receives information from the brain's cortex, as well as from the senses and countless cells of the body, and transforms them into the chemical messengers that trigger emotions, metabolic activity, and actions. Like a code, the hypothalamus interprets the quality of the breath and its rhythm from the Kundalini Yoga practice, along with the Shabad or Mantra, and in turn it activates the pineal and pituitary glands.[6]

BLESSINGS OF KUNDALINI RISING

Yogīs call the pineal gland the Thousand-Petaled Lotus, the seat of the soul. It sits at the center of the skull. When we chant in this uplifted state of Kundalini energy, those thousand petals start vibrating and stimulate the seventy-two Naadīs in the body, thus creating seventy-two thousand pulses of positive energy that course through the body. The yogīs say that as this happens, the lotus turns and rains nectar down upon us, cleansing the Chakras and filling us with blessings.[7]

The yogīs call the pituitary gland the Third Eye, and it acts as the seat of intuition. In Western anatomy, the pituitary gland works as a master gland for the body. It sits at the junction of the left and right optic nerves. When the hypothalamus stimulates the pituitary gland through chanting and Kundalini Yoga, we essentially affect our body through the neuroendocrine link in four areas: the autonomic nervous system, the endocrine system, the immune system, and the central nervous system. The autonomic nervous system includes our parasympathetic and sympathetic nervous systems. The parasympathetic nervous system enables us to relax. The sympathetic nervous system allows us to react quickly through fight or flight. Through the practice of Shabad Gurū, we strengthen our capacity to remain relaxed, centered, and calm no matter what. The endocrine system controls our moods and feelings of vitality and energy. Often people will report a sense of well-being or being "high" after chanting. The immune system keeps us healthy and resists diseases caused by stress. I believe we can create a healing response in our immune system by chanting the Shabad Gurū. Finally, through the practice of Shabad Gurū, we affect neurochemical communication in the central nervous system to increase our capacity to perceive and sense information from our environment. In short, we become more sensitive and perceptive.

> "What is Kundalini actually? You experience it when the energy of the glandular system combines with the nervous system to create such a sensitivity that the totality of the brain receives signals and integrates them. The person understands the effect of the effect in a sequence of the causes. In other words, man becomes totally and wholly aware. We call it the yoga of awareness. Just as all rivers end up in the ocean, all yogas end up raising the Kundalini in man."
>
> **YOGI BHAJAN**[8]

THE TEN BODIES

One morning a friend of mine brought her mother to our Aquarian Sādhanā practice. Her mother was elderly and could not sit on the floor; instead, she sat on a chair in the back of the room and participated whole-heartedly, even though she was unable to perform many of the physical movements. When the Sādhanā concluded, the woman had the most elevated expression on her face, and I stopped to talk to her before leaving to send my daughter off to school.

"That was such a beautiful experience!" she said with a bright smile while giving me a hug.

As I reflected on this experience later that day, I puzzled over the fact that her experience had been so good despite the fact that she had barely moved her body. For years I had associated the bliss of the Aquarian Sādhanā with the practice of doing yoga followed by chanting. A few months later I came to understand more when a Kundalini Yoga teacher explained the following: "We do not just have a physical body. We have ten bodies in all, and Kundalini Yoga works to heal, support, and transform them all."[9]

A trained Kundalini teacher learns to hold all ten bodies in consciousness while guiding the class, and therefore, someone can attend a Kundalini Yoga class and enjoy a totally blissful experience without using his or her physical body. The Aquarian Sādhanā also works to strengthen and foster an experience in all of these ten bodies, and I want you to know about them to better understand your physical, mental, and spiritual constitution (particularly if, like the woman I described above, you suffer from physical struggles on the earth plane).

For me personally, discovering these new dimensions of myself empowered and surprisingly pacified me. Needless to say, we are complex beings with a lot going on, and this yogic perspective gives color and shape to our unique existence and shows us a deeper reality than what meets the physical eye. Fortunately, we can engage in numerous yogic practices to support and strengthen each body; there's a Ten Bodies yoga set in appendix B for this very purpose. I highly recommend deepening your experience in Kundalini Yoga to discover all that's available to you. The Aquarian Sādhanā supports the healing, nourishment, and transformation of each of our bodies, and likewise our bodies become an important tool for deepening our practice.

Each of the ten Sikh Gurūs can help us strengthen each of our ten bodies through their subtle presence and also through a basic understanding of the events of their lives on this planet.[10] Below is a brief description of each of the bodies along with an example of how each Gurū can energetically help us.

First Body — Soul Body

If you want to get in touch with your soul, stop. Just stop, take a deep breath, and listen to the beat of your heart. This will connect you right away to your Soul Body, where you are simply present, pure, innocent, and real. When we vibrate within the excellence of the soul, we are not afraid.

Gurū Nānak, the first Sikh Gurū, can help you tap into your original nature, your self, and really just be who you are. He mastered this arena by starting a whole new *Dharma,* or spiritual path. He was in tune with the vibration of his soul, and although what he had to teach was considered radically different from the norm, people flocked to him because the essence of his soul connected with the essence of theirs.

Second Body—Negative Mind

The Second Body is the Negative Mind, which often gets a bad rap. This body holds the longing to belong and is therefore incredibly important. In the journey of belonging, this body watches out for pitfalls in the road, weaknesses in plans, and dangers of certain alliances. It measures the sum total of a situation and shows you the underside of it. When we get lost in this energy, we can become so overwhelmed with negative assessment that we freeze and become incapable of moving forward. However, if we remember that the essential purpose of the Negative Mind is the longing to belong, to be whole, to be in alignment, to be contained, and to be obedient to the greater Will of God, the Negative Mind becomes a powerful tool.

The energy of the Second Gurū, Gurū Angad, is helpful here, because he mastered the capacity to merge with the Divine Will come what may. His merger was so complete that Gurū Nānak named him "Angad," which means the limb, as in one's arm to the body. In this kind of merger with the Divine, no separation exists, and our Negative Mind becomes a much needed asset to serve the light within ourselves and everyone else.

Third Body—Positive Mind

I know some people with a strong Positive Mind; they can bring the mind into a state of expansiveness to feel all the possibilities. Being adept at the Negative Mind, I find a person with a robust Positive Mind fascinating, and even scary! Yet over the years, I have come to realize how invaluable a Positive Mind is—the capacity to go beyond fear and struggle, to say yes to life! Where does it stem from? Good self-esteem and a substantial navel point. These are essential in moving forward in life on all levels.

The Third Gurū, Gurū Amar Dās, illustrates the wonders of the Positive Mind. In the most difficult situations, we can rise above the fray sweetly, vigorously, and sure-footedly. Even as an old man, Gurū Amar Dās had the will to travel through a rainstorm at night to bring his Gurū fresh water from a river over two hours away. On foot! People thought he was crazy. Really, he was full of nothing but devotion, desiring to quench his Gurū's thirst with the best water he could find. This is how Gurū Amar Dās became the next Gurū. The obstacles in his path were no match for his Positive Mind.

Fourth Body—Neutral Mind

The Neutral Mind hears, assesses, evaluates, and understands the messages coming from the Positive and Negative Minds. It brings their energies to zero. Within this place of zero, we can take all of the information and act upon our consciousness. In the end, we only have our own consciousness to answer to: our own capacity to live in truth, live in the vibration of love, and rise in victory over the human intrigue, tumultuous ups and downs, and positives and negatives. How can we do this?

Compassion for ourselves, first and foremost. Compassion for all: for all the people in our lives, all the energies, positive and negative. Within this compassion, we unlock our heart to go deeper, and compassion shows the way to service. To serve the light of God within each and every situation is the key to liberation on this planet, step-by-step.

Neutrality is quiet. It just is. It's a bit lonely, even boring. When you are there, you are at the center of the Universe, with intuition and serenity as your best friends.

Gurū Rām Dās, the Fourth Gurū, can help us master our Neutral Mind. He lived an absolute life of service; he reached out to others before they even asked for help. He understood how to sit quietly, how to find the Neutral Mind, and how to allow the Universe to enact its play so that the ultimate truth could be illuminated to all.

Fifth Body—Physical Body

Mastery of the Physical Body is something that we can perhaps relate to. A healthy body generally means a longer life. That sounds good, right? Well, the yogīs take it a little deeper. They understand that it takes us 8.4 million lifetimes just to obtain this human birth, as we spent countless lives as stones, ferns, ants, squids, and on and on. And once we finally arrive at this human life, we may cycle through numerous human existences. Why? To learn our lessons, burn seeds of past bad karma, create new seeds of good karma, and finally find a spiritual path through which we can achieve union with God. The Physical Body offers an anchor, a way for us to go through this process and heal the rest of our bodies as well. To obtain mastery of the Physical Body, however, requires one step further. The way to mastery requires that our lives become examples of how to live in higher consciousness and how to sacrifice for the greater good of all.

They tortured Gurū Arjan, the fifth Gurū of the Sikhs, on a hot plate for five days and five nights. Instead of giving in to his torturers, he overcame the physical discomfort. The rulers of the time demanded that he conform to their ways. When one of his devotees pleaded to Gurū Arjan to give up, he refused, proclaiming that his life was about leaving an example for how to stand up for spirit and truth. In this same way, Jesus Christ mastered his Physical Body and dedicated it to the service of humanity. Those who obtain true mastery of the Physical Body leave a legacy for all time.

Sixth Body—Arcline

You know those pictures of saints with halos? Well, we all have one. And women have two! The yogīs call it the Arcline. The nucleus of our Aura, it extends from earlobe to earlobe above your brow and over your head. Each woman possesses a second Arcline that extends from nipple to nipple. Your Arcline directly links your physical body to the heavens. It is within the Arcline that we project our soul's prayer to where it eventually manifests on the planet. An identifying Mantra for the Arcline is "I am, I am." The first "I am" represents self-acceptance of who you are inside, and the second "I am" accepts that the Divine Self is all around you and knows that this is you as well. From this place of acceptance and clarity, the beautiful manifestation of the soul's prayer unfolds. Your vision of spirit can manifest on this planet just as it has for countless saints and inspirational leaders: Mother Theresa, the Dalai Lama, and Nelson Mandela, to name a few. All of them embodied spirit in the earthly realm in a very real way.

Gurū Hargobind, the Sixth Gurū, showed us how to master the Arcline. He had a jealous uncle who wanted his own son to be Gurū, so the uncle made various attempts on Gurū Hargobind's life. The young Hargobind prevailed with full joy and inner strength, the Mantra "I am, I am" resounding in his Arcline. Nothing could stop him. He became the Gurū after his father, Gurū Arjan, was tortured and killed by the Emperor. Gurū Hargobind established an army, trained his warriors, and within his lifetime not only created a martial defense against the Emperor, but also, with his intuitive nature, eventually established a positive and friendly alliance with that same Emperor. Through his clarity, he established the Akāl Takhat—the first mechanism for Sikhs to have a system of governance. All of this occurred against great odds, and the spirit of the people prevailed on the earth plane. It was not a miracle; it was a day-by-day, step-by-step process, all stemming from the incredible Arcline of Gurū Hargobind.

Seventh Body—the Aura

The Aura is the electromagnetic field around you. As mentioned before, the Aura is your first line of defense and is the result of your meditation and inner projection. We all have Auras that extend three to nine feet around us, and they intermingle with each other long before we shake hands. Because of this merging of vibrations, if we have a strong Aura, we can neutralize negative energy, and even emit healing energy. With weak Auras, however, we are subject to the influences of incoming energies. To strengthen the Aura, we need to meditate.

Gurū Har Rai, the Seventh Gurū, showed us the power of a strong Aura. In his lifetime, anyone who attempted to harm him failed without Gurū Har Rai even lifting a finger. Because of his strong, beautiful, and sweet vibration, the Universe adjusted itself to his vibration and served him.

Eighth Body—Prānic Body

It is through breath that we receive Prāna, the life force within each of us. Prāna brings us the gift of joy, courage, and elevation in life. When our Prānic Body is strong, we live fearlessly in the purity of who we are. When we tap into our inner Prāna, we find energy where there seemed to be none. One of the best ways to increase the health of our Prānic Body is through conscious breathing exercises called Prānayam.

Gurū Har Krishan, the Eighth Gurū, knew how to access Prāna. As a child of seven years of age, he healed hundreds of people who came to him during a plague. He healed them with Prāna through his hands. We all have Prāna inside us, and our daily practice helps to support the flow of this infinite energy source.

Ninth Body—Subtle Body

With the Subtle Body, we can relate to the greater play of life, see the unseen, and know the unknown. We can walk into a room full of people, assess the vibrations, and find a way to embody peace and serve everyone there. We can easily adjust in situations because we have already seen them in our meditations, and walking into life is a simple unfolding of something we already know. In this way, we learn quickly from life situations and obtain mastery in our endeavors. Life becomes a simple flow and play of the Divine. Experience of the Subtle Body comes through deep meditative practice.

The eighth Gurū, Gurū Har Krishan, named his successor while on his deathbed by only mentioning the town in which Gurū Teg Bahadur lived with the phrase, "Baba Bakala" (the wise father who lives in Bakala). After the eighth Gurū's death, many imposters set up shop in Bakala, all claiming to be Gurū, and it was a time of great confusion for the Sikhs. Instead of getting caught up in the fray, Gurū Teg Bahadur sat in deep meditation in a dark and secluded room underneath his home. The Gurū chose to put energy into his Subtle Body, to go to a deep place of inner mastery and serve his Sikhs from this place until the time of his inevitable discovery.

During this time it is said that a merchant captain caught in a fierce storm at sea called out for the Gurū's help. In his prayers he promised the Gurū five hundred gold coins. The ship miraculously made it to shore, and the captain—determined to pay the five hundred gold coins to his Gurū—set out to find him in Bakala. Discovering all of the imposters, the merchant captain tested them by offering each two gold coins. Each blessed the captain, accepted the two gold coins, and offered spiritual advice that had no depth. After seeing so many imposters, the captain became disheartened. He heard of one more holy man who lived just outside of town and set off to find him. It was in fact Gurū Teg Bahadur. The captain offered him two gold coins, and the Gurū said with a twinkle in his eyes, "Where are all five hundred coins? My shoulders are still sore from carrying your ship!" Once the captain heard this he fell at the Gurū's feet and then rushed up to the rooftop of the Gurū's house and loudly proclaimed, "I have found the True Gurū!" From this moment forward, Gurū Teg Bahadur was recognized by the Sikhs as the Gurū, and his life's work unfolded quickly and beautifully before him. He approached each situation with the energy of the Subtle Body, allowing his meditative presence to masterfuly serve, unravel cold hearts, and bring light to the truth.

Tenth Body—Radiant Body

The Radiant Body displays your nobility and courage. Kings and queens employ crowns in a similar way—they show the world their majesty. With a weak Radiant Body, we may fear standing out from the crowd and calling attention to ourselves. However, we must become familiar with our own nobility and courage—through these two elements, our soul sings its one true song. With our Radiant Body, we project ourselves with commitment and joy; everyone can feel it. People come to love and trust you, as they experience you to be committed, bright, and regal.

Gurū Gobind Singh, the Tenth Gurū, stood up to the Moghul Empire for spiritual and religious freedom of the Sikhs and people of all faiths in the region. Through his noble presence, people throughout the land felt protected, particularly the weak and innocent, even in the most challenging of times.

Eleventh Embodiment—Parallel Unisonness

The Eleventh Embodiment connects, supports, and orchestrates the vibrations of all ten bodies so that they align with the sound currents of the Divine. Yogi Bhajan said, "When the God in you, and the human in you are in parallel unisonness, then you are an eleven. You have no duality, you have divine vision, and the truth flows from you. You don't have to find anything outside of you. The jewels are all in you. You are rich inside; you have satisfaction and contentment."[11]

The Eleventh Embodiment exists as sound current. That is how the God in us and the human in us come into unity. In this process, we give ourselves completely—not to a great cause or someone we love, but to the impersonal Divine energy within us and within all beings. In this way we are "personally impersonal" as Yogi Bhajan liked to say. Manifesting in this way, anything is possible as long as we let go and let the Divine Will unfold.

For Sikhs, reciting the Eleventh Gurū, the Sirī Gurū Granth Sāhib, brings us into the Divine flow of wisdom and strengthens our Eleventh Embodiment. The elemental sounds of the Eleventh Gurū carry a flow of consciousness and wisdom, imparting this energy to the reader, even when we don't know the meaning of the words. Jap Jī, in stage two of the Aquarian Sādhanā, is the first composition of this sacred text. Daily recitation of Jap Jī strengthens our Eleventh Embodiment.

THE CHAKRA SYSTEM AND THE TEN BODIES IN THE AQUARIAN SĀDHANĀ

I have learned that I cannot separate my spiritual practice from my day-to-day life. True liberation comes not only through our meditation practice, but also through our thoughts, our choices, our speech, and the actions we choose in every moment of every day. I recommend using the Chakra system and the understanding of the ten bodies to evaluate the areas of your life that need support, as well as those areas in which you feel steady and strong. Becoming familiar with your Chakras and ten bodies in this way will help you understand life changes better and lead you into increased health, balance, and strength. The Aquarian Sādhanā will undoubtedly support you in this process. As Yogi Bhajan reminds us, "The whole world around you will be beautiful if you understand that you are you. In all walks of your life remember you are you. 'I am, I am.' That is the Mantra. The Kundalini and Kundalini Yoga are very natural elements that rapidly make you what you are already and bring you to the practical experience of infinity."[12]

~ Chapter Four ~

ALTAR OF THE SELF

Stage One: Preparing for the Aquarian Sādhanā

ਮਨੁ ਕਰਿ ਮਕਾ ਕਿਬਲਾ ਕਰਿ ਦੇਹੀ ॥

man kar makā kibalā kar dayhī.

Let your mind be Mecca, and your body the temple of worship.

ਬੋਲਨਹਾਰੁ ਪਰਮ ਗੁਰੁ ਏਹੀ ॥੧॥

bolanahār param gur ayhī. ‖ 1‖

Let the Supreme Gurū be the One who speaks. ‖1‖

ਕਹੁ ਰੇ ਮੁਲਾਂ ਬਾਂਗ ਨਿਵਾਜ ॥

kah(u) ray mulā(n) bāng nivāj.

O Mullah, utter the call to prayer.

ਏਕ ਮਸੀਤਿ ਦਸੈ ਦਰਵਾਜ ॥੧॥ ਰਹਾਉ ॥

ayk masīt dasai daravāj. ‖ 1‖ rahā-u.

The one mosque has ten doors. ‖1‖Pause‖

KABĪR JĪ, *SIRĪ GURŪ GRANTH SĀHIB JĪ*[1]

In the first step of the Aquarian Sādhanā, we prepare for the practice itself. Although preliminary, this stage is just as important as any of the others, as the steps we take here bring us joy, empowerment, grounding, royalty, and peace. This chapter focuses on creating a place to meditate and following the yogī's wake-up routine. Truly our spiritual practice begins with the first breath of life, and the yogīs say that sleeping, waking, eliminating, bathing, and dressing are just as important as the actual act of meditating.

A PLACE TO MEDITATE

I have found that one way to really shift the energy of your life is to create a sacred space where you meditate every day. We have a place to cook our food, we have a place to sleep, and we have a place to take a shower, so we need a place dedicated to our meditation as well. Making one declares to visitors, to your family, and to your own mind that spirit is a priority in your life. The power of chanting and meditating affects not only spiritual matters, but physical matters as well. In fact, as we meditate in a space day after day, the floor, walls, and surrounding objects are literally permeated with the vibrations of our practice. Whether or not our family or neighbors join us, the energy of our meditation can be felt on a subtle level.

Begin by creating an altar for yourself, something you can focus on during your meditation; it can include a candle, inspiring pictures, prayers, and other uplifting objects. I have found throughout the years that by keeping my altar neat, clean, and dust-free, with a few fresh flowers, it truly enlivens my meditation practice. Remember, yoga means union. As householders, it's not just what we do in our yoga and meditation practice that matters, but also how we take that practice out into our daily lives. In a way, our entire home acts as an altar space. We can also consider our workspace in a similar way. When we are on the phone with someone who's having a hard time, we can glance at something sacred, perhaps a flower, and remember to take a deep breath, and this simple act embodies our presence over the phone with authenticity and comfort. Of course, life gets messy; we don't have to keep our space picture-perfect all of the time. I'm just encouraging you to create the intention of sacred vibration in your environment.

As our morning practice begins, we become more tuned in and sensitive to energies that support the environments that Spirit thrives in, and likewise we become aware of those things that don't. Perhaps a particular picture on the wall does not offer supportive energy. Perhaps you need to open a window. Find out what makes you and your Spirit rejoice.

In the past year, my family and I moved several times in search of a home. In our first move, we had not decided on a place for our family Gurdwārā, or place of worship. For several months, the Sirī Gurū Granth Sāhib, our sacred text, sat in a box on top of a stack of other boxes in one of our rooms. Granted, it was a fancy box, but a box nonetheless. Finally, we determined where our meditation space would be, set our Gurdwārā up, and, as is the Sikh custom to celebrate the opening of a Gurdwārā, we took a Hukam from the Sirī Gurū Granth Sāhib. From the text's nearly fifteen hundred pages, one selects the reading after meditating, opening the book to whatever page is meant to be read. I can't remember the exact phrasing of this Hukam, but it went something like this: "You had me high in the sky. Now you have brought me down to the earth, and I have a home. The Gurū has been installed."

That blew me away. I heard the voice of the Divine speaking directly to me, and I realized how clearly the presence of the Gurū was with us. The last time we moved, I set up the Gurdwārā right away, not wanting to keep the Gurū waiting.

SOMETHING TO SIT ON

When you meditate, try to sit on something made from natural fiber. The yogīs sat on sheepskin. You can do that too, but keep in mind that the yogīs obtained these skins with a lot of attention and care. When they meditated on the skin of an animal, they always prayed for the animal's soul. These days it is difficult to find skins taken from animals in a conscious way. So, I recommend using wool or cotton mats. It's nice to have a little padding, but not too much, and try to get something that doesn't slip. Natural fibers are much better for the nervous system, so if you have a favorite yoga mat made of synthetic material, cover it with something natural. I recommend sitting on the same mat day after day to infuse it with your practice. Especially if you travel a lot, take something familiar with you to sit on. Your mat becomes your home away from home.

I also recommend using a shawl to blanket yourself with during deep relaxation and to cover your spine while meditating. Through the practice, we generate a lot of energy in the spinal cord, and covering ourself helps us to better contain that energy. If you are in a warm climate I suggest covering at least the base of your spine with a thin shawl.

EARLY MORNING PRACTICE TIPS

ਅੰਮ੍ਰਿਤ ਵੇਲਾ ਸਚੁ ਨਾਉ ਵਡਿਆਈ ਵੀਚਾਰੁ ॥

amrit vaylā sach nā-u vadi-ā-ī vīchār.

In the Amrit Vaylā, the ambrosial hours before dawn, chant the True Name,
and contemplate His Glorious Greatness.

ਕਰਮੀ ਆਵੈ ਕਪੜਾ ਨਦਰੀ ਮੋਖੁ ਦੁਆਰੁ ॥

karamī āvai kaparā nadarī mokh du-ār.

By the karma of past actions, the robe of this physical body is obtained.
By His Grace, the Gate of Liberation is found.

ਨਾਨਕ ਏਵੈ ਜਾਣੀਐ ਸਭੁ ਆਪੇ ਸਚਿਆਰੁ ॥੪॥

nānak ayvai jānī-ai sabh āpay sachiār. || 4||

O Nānak, know this well: the True One Himself is All. || 4||

GURŪ NĀNAK, *FOURTH PAURĪ OF JAP JĪ*[2]

We practice this Sādhanā in the Amrit Vaylā, the "Nectar Hour" between four and seven in the morning. Yogi Bhajan taught that this is the time period that is an optimal time to meditate on God because of the sun's angle in addition to the fact that the world is usually quiet.[3] It's also the time when our subconscious downloads itself. The subconscious acts as the storehouse of all of the feelings, emotions, and impressions we have yet to consciously heal or process. When we do not cleanse our subconscious, it can rule our lives. Instead of living from our inner truth, we act out from inner burdens and past wounds or traumas. The subconscious desperately wants to download itself, and meditation helps us achieve this. I remember Yogi Bhajan comparing the process to cleaning a toilet bowl.

During the Sādhanā you may experience an increase in thoughts. Don't worry about this; the trick is to not get caught in the thoughts, but to allow the technology of the sacred recitations, yoga, and chanting to work for you and heal you on a deep level. The practice cleanses you by pulling out the negative energy of the subconscious like a vortex, and you can measure that process by the intensity of your thoughts. As the subconscious gets purified, thoughts increase, like the swish of water in the toilet bowl as the brush does its job. Stay with the Mantra and the breath, go deeper, and let God clean you out. You can go deeper and deeper, into a state beyond thoughts, the Anahat.

That being said, some thoughts—"little gems"—arise here and there like messages from God and Gurū; some of these thoughts have uplifted me and brought a lot of joy into my life. These little gems are easy to identify because they are usually accompanied by a deep breath. I often receive ideas about work-related issues that I am grappling with, ideas that take me out of the struggle and show me a universal perspective and enlightened solution to the issue at hand. Yet even small, mundane thoughts can be important, too; for example, maybe you suddenly remember that you have a carpool that day. Honor these worldly thoughts, too. I don't know how many times I've experienced thoughts like these during Sādhanā that saved me in some way. I learned from my father to keep a little notebook handy for such instances.

However, keep in mind that the Sādhanā is not a time to make business plans, decide what you are going to do with the kids that day, or what you will make for breakfast. All of those things are important, of course, but you can take care of them later; this is the time for you and your love relationship with God. Preserve that with your intention. Like me, you'll get around to preparing your daughter for school, shopping, going to the bank, and all of the other things we have to do on the earth, but you'll do it with your whole self—intact, cleansed, and lighter.

Okay, so now you may be asking how in the world does one wake up so early? Aside from a few incredible yogīs and other people who can exist with hardly any sleep, most of us need a proper amount of sleep to function well and stay healthy. If you don't know what that amount is for yourself, I encourage you to research it and figure it out. Doing so will help you engage in the Sādhanā with vitality and stability. And, yes, it most likely means going to bed early. As Benjamin Franklin said, "Early to bed, early to rise, makes a man healthy, wealthy, and wise."[4] I couldn't agree more! However, I suffered from sleep deprivation for years and had trouble creating a consistent Sādhanā practice. I would start off gung ho, but after a few weeks I'd find myself exhausted and getting sick to the degree that I had to modify or shorten my practice. Finally, my husband and I decided to go to bed when our daughter did, much earlier in the evening, and this is how I arrived at a steady and sustainable Sādhanā practice, the benefits of which have inspired me to write this manual. Of course, going to bed early means giving up some things like socializing during the evening, but I've come to discover the changes are worth it: love still exists, life still exists, and miracles still exist the rest of the hours of the day, in even more richness and fullness when I fulfill my soul. It's a simple matter of shifting your life. People get used to the fact that you go to bed early. In fact, as you tap into Spirit more and more, you acclimate to the change and may even find yourself waking up minutes before the alarm goes off, your whole self engaged and ready to go.

If you live in a place where the light changes are more extreme and the angle of the sun's rays hitting the earth are a bit different (like, say, Alaska), or you simply can't adjust to waking up early, please remember that the primary point here is to have your time with the Divine before the day starts. I invite you to start the journey of carving out this precious time for yourself even if it may not look exactly like the traditional Amrit Vaylā.

A KUNDALINI YOGĪ'S WAY TO START THE DAY

To recognize the royalty within you and truly experience bliss in the body, the following are some simple yet totally effective morning yogic techniques to help you enjoy living in your body temple.

Clearing Out Mucus

Yogīs everywhere brush their teeth before meditating because it cleans out bacteria from the mouth. Additionally, after you finish brushing your teeth, use your toothbrush to clean your tongue all the way back to your throat. This will make you gag a little bit, which helps clear mucus from your respiratory system.[5]

Elimination and Diet

After you have brushed your teeth, drink a large glass of warm water. If your digestion is good and you are getting enough sleep, at this point you can have a bowel movement. As yogīs, we try to have a bowel movement at the beginning of each day, to let out what was put in yesterday before we consume more food today. Plus, having an empty gut for meditation is a blissful experience.

If you eat meat, you might have trouble making a bowel movement every morning because meat is hard to digest. In this way, a vegetarian lifestyle is quite pragmatic. Of course, we can look at it energetically as well: when an animal is killed and we eat it, we take in that animal's karmic energy of fear it felt at the moment of death. Every energetic influence—whether we generate it or digest it—either contributes or takes away from the sanctity and purity of our inner space.

That being said, every person is different. Even if you don't eat meat, you may have difficulty defecating, and lots of people don't have a bowel movement every morning. To achieve this might take a lot of time and substantial dietary changes for your body type. If you wish to explore further, I recommend the science of Ayurveda, a health system from India, as it has helped me a lot in this regard; please review the resources section for more information.

Taking Care of Your Hair

As I've mentioned before, Kundalini means Lock of the Beloved. Needless to say, hair is sacred in the Kundalini Yoga tradition. From an early age, my mother taught me to attend to my hair with great attention, and I love the feeling of combing my hair in the morning with love and care. In this tradition, we wash our hair every seventy-two hours, and I find that following this guideline increases my mental clarity. The recommendation is to wash your hair and let the sun dry it naturally. Try to use a natural fiber comb, preferrably made of wood, or a brush with natural bristles, and comb it in the morning to support the Kundalini rising. The yogīs see hair as a natural conduit of solar energy: combing it and placing it in a spiral shape at the top of the head brings all of this subtle light energy to work. At night we comb the hair down to promote relaxation. You can also apply natural oil to the tips.

Our body hair helps to balance our electromagnetic field and acts as an antenna for our Aura. That's why we pay attention to all of our hair, including under our arms and on our legs, and we don't shave it. The hair naturally grows in areas of the body that house major glands, and the hair helps to protect the hormone functions of these areas. Additionally, hair takes a lot of protein to create, so when we cut or shave our hair, we require our body to use a lot more protein—protein that we could otherwise use for other important health functions. Yogi Bhajan's teachings tell us that a man's beard covers the pranic nerve in the chin that is controlled by the moon. He needs this protection, whereas a woman's nervous system can handle the effect of the moon.[6]

Cold Shower

This is hard for a lot of people, but don't skip this paragraph! Cold showers offer a lot of benefits: As the cold water hits our skin, blood rushes up to open the capillaries. Then the blood moves to our internal organs as a means of protection, and this process releases excess heat from the body. When blood moves this way, it becomes oxygenated and flushes the entire body, which benefits our skin, organs, and lymphatic and endocrine systems. The cold water, especially when accompanied with massage, really aids your skin and complexion. The whole experience totally recharges the nervous system; it also increases the parasympathetic reflex: our capacity to handle stress successfully.[7] In my experience, taking cold showers brings a steadiness to my energy, and they help me remain uplifted and peaceful throughout the whole day. Here's how I suggest taking a cold shower for the maximum benefit:

1. Rub almond oil, or another kind of pure and natural oil, on your body. Ayurveda advises to only apply to your skin that which you are willing to eat (this cuts out moisturizers with synthetic scents, which most of us would never think of drinking). In some ways, our skin is our most important organ, as it acts as our first line of defense. As you massage oil into your skin, know that you are doing something loving for your skin, for your energy, and for yourself.

2. Put on some cotton shorts. In India we call these "kacheras." These shorts can be especially helpful for people living in cold climates or for those who have a sensitivity to cold water. But primarily kacheras protect the thighbone from direct contact with cold water. As the thighbone regulates calcium levels along with your parathyroid, it should ideally remain protected from direct contact with the cold.

3. Get into the shower and go for it! Most likely you may have some sort of verbal expletive! This is good. For maximum benefit, try an uplifting Mantra like *Wāhegurū*. *Wāh* means great! or wow!; *he* means here and now; and *gurū*, of course, refers to the One who brings us from darkness to light. Chant this repeatedly as the shower inspires you.

4. Start by putting your extremities (hands, feet, arms, and legs) in first and massage them until they are warm, before proceeding with the rest of your body. Massage yourself all over as the cold water hits your skin. Massage under your armpits, as these house major nerve centers, and women in particular should massage their breasts for general breast health. As you continue to massage your body, the oil that you put on your skin earlier gets repelled by the water, so it sinks deeper into your skin. This has a great moisturizing effect.

5. When you finish, dry off with a towel and give yourself a good rub. This takes off any dead skin and further invigorates the nervous system.

6. Get dressed!

A few additional notes about the cold shower: Use your discretion, but it's recommended to avoid a cold shower when you are in the heavy part of your moon cycle. Also, don't take one if you are seven months pregnant or more (although it's great for your baby before that time). You may also want to refrain if you have a cold or flu. And, of course, some people just don't have the constitution for cold showers in general. Don't worry if it doesn't work for you, but I'm convinced of the benefits if you can stand it!

Dressing for Meditation

Yogi Bhajan taught us to get dressed in clothes that are uplifting and feel good as we do our daily discipline. Growing up, I usually just rolled into Sādhanā in my pajamas because it resembled how my parents brought me in, all wrapped up in blankets asleep! However, when I read Yogi Bhajan's teachings about consciously dressing for Sādhanā some thirty years later, I gave it a shot. I loved it. I found it an ingenious way to convince my mind that something special was underway for me. It uplifted my whole outlook on the practice and thus deepened my experience in a very real way.

Of course, the Sādhanā includes yoga, so wear something comfortable that you can easily move in. As noted before, Yogi Bhajan emphasized wearing natural fabrics such as cotton, silk, and wool in our practice and in our daily lives. He also taught us that wearing white helps us to tap into the positive energy of the universe. Because white contains all of the colors of the spectrum, it naturally promotes acceptance and universal love. In addition, white acts as a reflector, so it protects us from negative energy. When we meditate a lot, we become more sensitive to the energy of people, environments, and situations, so having this capacity to reflect rather than absorb becomes helpful. Finally, white enhances and projects the Aura.[8]

Although I have told you virtually everything *to* put on, please *don't* put on your socks! When we practice Kundalini Yoga and meditation, it is best to have the feet uncovered. The feet and hands have a large concentration of nerve endings that directly communicate to our nervous system. As Dr. Hari Simran Singh says, "The nerve endings are our antennas into our experience and covering them muffles the messages. Feeling the elements in the extremities is an important aspect of the total Kundalini Yoga experience. The wind on the skin, the circulation of fluid, even sound (vibration) is subtly heard in the nerve endings."[9]

Head Covering

Yogi Bhajan recommended that we cover our head for the Aquarian Sādhanā. You can use several different creative head-covering styles (a few are illustrated below), but try to employ natural fibers. The teachings tell us that keeping the hair uncut, coiled at the top of the head

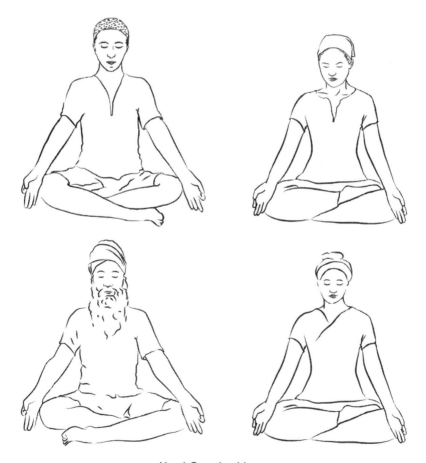

Head-Covering Ideas

and covered with a natural fiber in the form of a turban, supports the downward movement of solar energy from the top of the head and can activate the rise of the Kundalini energy at the base of the spine. Although this is the ideal scenario for a Kundalini yogī and a Sikh, there are other acceptable head-covering options for people with different lifestyle choices. Someone with short hair, wearing another head-covering option besides a turban, will still undoubtedly experience something powerful and transformative in the Aquarian Sādhanā.

In my own experience, I find that chanting activates the higher Chakras. Having a head covering protects and contains the energy as this process occurs, and allows it to stabilize for a more sustained experience that lasts throughout the day. Yogi Bhajan taught us how to wrap a turban and explained that the turban stimulates meridian points on the skull that give us a cranial adjustment as an aid to remaining alert and balanced. For me, my turban is my crown. As I wrap it, I chant. I wear it for my practice and then also throughout the day. Through all challenges of life, I have a reminder to remain in my grace and strength. One look in the mirror, and I am reminded of who I am.[10]

~ Chapter Five ~

MEDITATION OF THE SOUL

Stage Two: Jap Jī

ਨਾਮੁ ਸੁਣੈ ਨਾਮੁ ਸੰਗ੍ਰਹੈ ਨਾਮੇ ਲਿਵ ਲਾਵਉ ॥

nām suṇay nām sangrahai nāmay liv lāvu.

I hear the Nām (the Name of God), and I gather in the Nām;
I am lovingly attuned to the Nām.

GURŪ ARJAN, *SIRĪ GURŪ GRANTH SĀHIB JĪ*[1]

As we sit down to engage in the Aquarian Sādhanā, we begin by reciting the entire Jap Jī, which you will find in appendix A. The main purpose of this chapter is to give you a history of Jap Jī, explain its healing effects, describe how we recite it in the Aquarian Sādhanā, and suggest other meditative practices to accompany this sacred text. If you'd like more guidance, please order a copy of *Meditation of the Soul: Jap Jī Daily Practice and Learning Tool* (you can find out more about it in the resources section).

ORIGINS OF JAP JĪ

In 1469, Gurū Nānak was born in a town called Talwandi (now a part of Pakistan). At birth, the local astrologer predicted that he would become a renowned saint and teacher. Nānak was born at a time with a dominating caste system, ill treatment of women, and intense separation and strife between Hindus and Muslims. To the dismay and frustration of his father, Nānak enjoyed playing with children of different religions and castes, spending time with yogīs in the forest, and meditating. His father would have preferred that he conform to the normal ways of the day.

As a young man, Nānak lived a traditional life for his time—he married, had two sons, and worked in a government grain shop. Every morning, Nānak would rise before the sun and bathe in the cold river near his home and then meditate before going to work. On one particular morning, Nānak submerged into the river but did not come up again; a search ensued, but they never found his body in the river or anywhere nearby on shore. After three days and with tremendous sadness, his family and fellow villagers prepared for his funeral. At that moment, Nānak emerged from the river and proclaimed, "There is no Hindu, and there is no Muslim." He meant that we cannot separate ourselves from the Divine light within each of us; he meant that we all come from one source, Ek Ong Kār, and that it was this that created all of us. Nānak then offered everyone in attendance a chant, the Mūl Mantra, which is the third chant in the Aquarian Sādhanā.

Later, Nānak described his underwater experience (later termed "Jal Samādhi," or merger with the One in the water). He said he went to "Sach Kand" or the "True Home," where it became clear to him as a directive of the Divine that he should dedicate his life to teaching. This is when he became known as Gurū Nānak. He dressed like a cross between a Hindu and a Muslim and set out with his disciple, Mardana, to teach.[2] They traveled on foot everywhere; there are countless stories describing how Gurū Nānak touched people's lives.

Here's one of them: There was a queen named Noor Shah who practiced sorcery. She liked to capture innocent travelers and cast spells on them. This gave her a lot of pleasure, and she especially enjoyed capturing holy men because it made her feel very powerful.

Gurū Nānak and Mardana were travelling near Noor Shah's palace and stopped to rest. Mardana asked if he could go to town to look for food as he was quite hungry. Gurū Nānak gave his consent. As Mardana approached the town, he came to the palace, and some of the queen's female attendants were delighted to see what appeared

66

to be a holy man approaching, seeing him as a worthy prize for their queen. Offering him tea and sweets, they lured the hungry Mardana inside for a promised meal, where in fact he came under the spell of the queen. Thinking that he was a goat, Mardana got on all fours and began to bleat helplessly. Somewhere deep inside, he called out to Gurū Nānak, who heard his plea.

Gurū Nānak came straight away to the palace. Seeing a second holy man, the queen was beside herself with excitement. She tried all of her spells on Gurū Nānak, but to no avail—everything she tried to inflict came back on her. Finally, Noor Shah fell at his feet, sobbing and requesting to be his disciple, to learn his magic. Gurū Nānak encouraged her to give her riches to the poor, stop manipulating people with black magic, and chant God's Name.[3]

After profoundly affecting the lives of Queen Noor and thousands of others, Gurū Nānak moved on, but he remained quite present through his words. He wrote poems and kept them at his waist in a little book; the poems were easy to memorize because of their wonderful rhythm, rhyme, and deep meaning. Eventually a number of these were brought together, and under Gurū Nānak's guidance they became known as Jap Jī.

THE EFFECTS OF RECITATION

"What is Jap Jī, do you know? Jap Jī is a permutation and combination of the sound current to bring balance and relevancy to the productivity of the neurons in the brain via the hypothalamus. And it sets the pattern to experience infinity."

YOGI BHAJAN[4]

Gurū Nānak left us a pathway to his merger with the One, his Jal Samādhi, with Jap Jī. When I recite these words, I feel in a flow of something larger than myself. I don't want to be doing anything else, and I experience ease, peace, and great comfort in the words. When I finish, I feel lighter in my mind or perhaps in my brain. It's kind of like having a mechanic work on the engine of your car (the brain): it takes a lot of hammering, unscrewing, and poking. The work comes from the pulsation of the words as they reverberate in the cave of the mouth and then move into the neural pathways.

Yogi Bhajan taught so much about Jap Jī; I'm sure I will spend my entire lifetime making new discoveries of his teachings on this subject alone. Here's one of my favorites: As we recite the Jap Jī, it adjusts all of the five elements in the body—earth, air, fire, water, and ether—along with all eight Chakras. Five multiplied by eight equals forty, and there are forty stanzas in the Jap Jī that represent the steps of consciousness on our journey to merger with the One. Yogi Bhajan gave us a view into how this works. When we recite the first Paurī (the Mūl Mantra), we adjust the ether element and the eighth Chakra. After reciting the final stanza, we have adjusted the first Chakra and the earth element.[5]

Here's a more personal example of how Jap Jī can work on us: I had been in the studio for a few days recording my vocals for an album. My producer, Thomas, is from Germany; he's a dedicated yogī himself and brilliant composer and musician. Maybe it's the German in him, but he's usually totally tapped into accurate rhythm. He's a compassionate guy, but the past few days had been tense and trying for both of us. For whatever reason, my lyrical rhythm was a little off, and we seemed to be missing some sort of sparkle in the whole process.

That morning we prepared to record the fifth Paurī of Jap Jī. We had already recorded the music for the track, and now it was time for my final vocals. I sat in the darkness and silence of the recording room, breathing and praying, "Oh God, please let me be a channel. Please allow these words of Gurū Nānak to come through and serve humanity." I waited until my fears quieted, and I arrived in a place of surrender. Then I told Thomas I was ready.

As my first take began, I sank right into the rhythm of the words, feeling a deep sense of comfort and belonging. At some point I experienced a shift in consciousness; I no longer felt important, and I stopped blocking the energy. It felt like the presence of Gurū Nānak himself: I experienced the openness of the Cosmos where eternal love reigns supreme. There was nothing left for me to do but sing.

The rest of the recording session unfolded with ease, totally blessed by this experience. I realized later that after years and years of reciting Jap Ji, the words had become familiar friends. I could access their wisdom and peace any time I wanted. And if I ever needed balancing or realigning, Jap Ji would always be right there to help. The particular track I'm referring to is called "So Mai Visar Na Jaa-ee." You can find information about it and the other musical tracks from Jap Ji that I have recorded in the resources section. As noted earlier, you have a recitation of Jap Ji included with this book called *Jap Ji Meditation*.

Jap means repeat, and *Ji* means soul. Through repeating Jap Ji daily, we attune our soul to the universal conciousness that Gurū Nānak embodied. This amazing poem teaches us how to live in consciousness on this planet, and it explores topics such as deep listening, surrender, faith, and ways to access the energy of infinity within us. Jap Ji also encourages us to practice from a place of love, sit within the polarities of the Universe in complete balance and serenity, and apply ourselves wholeheartedly to spiritual discipline. As we recite it with each repetition, we teach ourselves through its vibration; we don't even have to know the meaning. On a cellular level, we are shifting the vibratory frequency of our being.

> "We must do ourselves a favor. Gurū Nānak gave us Jap Ji.
> Jap means repeated, reciprocal creative power. Jap means
> when we recite and what we recite, it takes mind, body, and
> soul to recite; Jap requires consciousness, intelligence, and
> personality; it requires soul, mind, and body. Ji means the
> soul, the inner self, the eternal self, the excellent self, the
> infinite self, that is called Ji. Ji energy is what the universal
> energy is, and Gurū Nānak gave you Jap of the Ji,
> that's why the name is Jap Ji. It is recitation of that Ji,
> it is called multiple soul, it's called infinite soul."
>
> **YOGI BHAJAN**[6]

This is not a quiet meditative practice! It requires you to Jap, actively! As you recite, I encourage you to try it in the original Gurmukhī, a healing language. By using Gurmukhī, you reset the neural patterns of your brain to more perfectly match the consciousness patterns that Gurū Nānak experienced.

For this reason, although you can use the provided recording to learn the pronunciation, I highly recommend that you use your own voice for this practice. Eventually, when you feel comfortable, you can turn off the recording and just hear your own voice or the voices of your community. Doing so, you activate a chamber in your skull where the resonance of your voice will begin to form. This is an essential part of the healing process. It must be your voice, and you must have the capacity to hear it.

When I was eighteen, I spent a few months in Amritsar, a holy city in Northern India. We stayed across the street from the Golden Temple, a beautiful temple made of marble on the inside and gold on the outside that sits in a sparkling pool of water. It sits in an enclosed plaza that creates a serene space in the midst of a busy city. We went there to meditate every day, and I found complete happiness in this blissful routine. One day during my visit, an adventurous friend who loves to explore took me to another Gurdwārā in the center of town. After a dusty rickshaw ride, we found ourselves in the middle of an overwhelmingly busy street. I could not imagine that any place of worship could exist near all the shops, cows, honking horns, and throngs of people. I followed my friend as she wove in and out of the madness and, suddenly, we popped into an open doorway. As I crossed the threshold, I realized we had entered the grounds of the Gurdwārā, a quiet courtyard nestled in the busy city with shelves for shoes. Removing my shoes, I entered the temple sanctuary, and it was packed: five hundred people all sitting side by side, all of them reciting Jap Ji. The vibration came pouring over us. Voices like waves of the ocean passed over me, and I could feel them healing every cell and fiber of my being. My friend whispered to me through the waves of sound that they recited Jap Ji repeatedly every Sunday. I perceived that they had been doing it for so long that the vibration of the recitation took over the space and my heart. I bowed my head to the Sirī Gurū Granth Sāhib, and sat down and bathed, literally bathed, in the bliss. It was the magic of Jap Ji.

TIPS FOR AN UPLIFTING EXPERIENCE OF JAP JĪ

Over the years, I have picked up the following tips that have really uplifted my Jap Jī practice that I'd like to share with you.

Posture

When you read Jap Jī, sit with a nice straight spine on something comfortable that supports your hips. Hold your booklet, or whatever you are reading Jap Jī from, in such a way that you can sit up straight. When we recite while sitting erect, we engage and stimulate all the Chakras along the spinal cord. The vibration of the words enters each Chakra and creates a spin that sends the healing waves of the words throughout your body through your seventy-two Naadīs, or healing channels. As I suggested before, wear a shawl or blanket as needed to make sure that your spine remains warm during this process.

Pronunciation

It's a great idea to work on your pronunciation. As the sacred words pass through your mouth, the tongue taps the roof of your mouth and sends messages to your hypothalamus. The healing vibration of these words then affects you positively in a physical way, so improving your pronunciation will amplify this entire healing process. If you find yourself reading along with Jap Jī and becoming a little cross-eyed, I invite you to sit within the confusion and try to suspend your understanding of regular reality. Something special is happening. Keep the focus, stay with it, and perfect it. Reading a sacred language in a meditative way can become a *Drishtī*, a yogic eye focus. This is a tool for shifting one's consciousness and experiencing great bliss.

Breath

Please remember to breathe during the recitation! The recitation itself is a breathing system that brings in Prāna, the life force of the Universe. In order to make the system work, however, you need to put breath into it. I suggest taking moments to inhale and exhale expansively as it feels natural to you. Try to remain full and connected to a sense of abundance with your breath as you recite.

Rhythm

Keep a steady rhythm with the recitation. Often Jap Ji is recited in musical form, and it is with music that Gurū Nānak conveyed many of his teachings. That was no accident. In music we are blessed with rhythm, and we create a meditative spin that takes the mind into a trancelike state. In the recitation of Jap Ji, if you apply this basic rhythm principle it will greatly deepen your experience.

Meaning

I encourage you to read the translation of Jap Ji as often as you can. There is such incredible wisdom in these words! Although you don't have to know the meaning to receive the benefit of the words, I find that understanding the meaning as much as I can, reflecting on it, and applying it to my life brings wonderful results. As well, the meaning of these beautiful words brings comfort and calm.

Voice

Although you can use the recording provided with this book or the one included in *Meditation of the Soul: Jap Ji Daily Practice and Learning Tool* to learn Jap Ji, I sincerely hope you will come to recite it on your own. (This learning tool is something we created for people who wish to go deeper in the study of Jap Ji.) Real change comes through your own participation: your words and your energy. Keep the tune simple for yourself and others. Some mornings you may have a lot of time, and so you can recite Jap Ji slowly, really getting the vibration of it. Other mornings you may feel more hurried, and on those days you can recite more quickly and still benefit as long as you make an effort to pronounce the words correctly.

Head

By covering your head, you contain the vibration of the recitation in your body. Keeping that energy inside allows you to access it during the recitation, and then it gets stabilized so that you have a chance to merge with it and allow it to guide you through your day. Covering the head also honors the tradition from which Jap Ji comes and will bring forth the energy of all those devotees who have recited it before you.

Ten Bodies

Because recitation repatterns our brain neurons, it can be a rather intense process. Often we respond to intensity by becoming mentally distracted—an inexperienced reciter can become overwhelmed and frustrated, an experienced one can carry on logical streams of thought during the recitation, which also leads to disconnection. Unfortunately, we lose most of the benefits when distracted.

To allow the process to unfold gracefully and maintain a meditative state so that healing can occur, recite Jap Ji from all of your bodies! Let your toes tingle in the recitation! Feel the subtlety of your being—feel it in your Aura, your breath, your Arcline. Don't be afraid to expand. Once you allow yourself this expansion, you can sit neutrally within the process of the brain transformation occurring and actually hold the energy in a stabilizing manner so that the total and complete transformation can occur. Expand out to the unexpected places of your being to remain focused on the task at hand.

TANTRIC-STYLE RECITATION OF JAP JI

ਦਿਵਸੁ ਰਾਤਿ ਦੁਇ ਦਾਈ ਦਾਇਆ ਖੇਲੈ ਸਗਲ ਜਗਤੁ ॥

divas rāt du-i dā-ī dā-i-ā khaylai sagal jagat.

Day and night are the two nurses, in whose lap all the world is at play.

GURŪ NĀNAK, *SALOK OF JAP JĪ*[1]

As Gurū Nānak teaches us, the world is at play between two polarities: day and night, sun and moon, woman and man. If we maintain balance between these polarities, we will feel as at home with them as a little child in the lap of her mother or father or the "Divine Parent." Let's take a closer look at the polarities of women and men.

In Kundalini Yoga we often refer to the woman as moon and to the man as sun. What does the moon do? She reflects the energy of the sun. She reigns supreme in the cool of the dark night—vast, open, and ready to receive from a boundless inner space. The moon is grace, kindness, and ultimate strength. She travels through her cycle every twenty-eight days, and as the moon takes on different shapes, she learns to love the changes as her grace guides her through them. She contains the energy of her family within her circular shape, and her presence provides warmth and coziness.

What does the sun do? He projects his rays outward, steady and constant, from his internal connection to the Divine, shining without fear into the unknown. And just as the woman waxes every fourteen days and then wanes for the same length of time, Yogi Bhajan taught us that the man waxes within fourteen breaths and wanes for the same. The length of his cycle is only roughly two minutes, depending on his length of breath. According to the yogīs, he is undergoing a massive energetic change in a very short period of time. Just as we can't detect the individual movement of a hummingbird's wings, man moves too fast for us to percieve his changes. Although he appears steady, it takes a lot of strength to hold that steadiness. Just as the sun rises every day, so does man. We gather around the warmth of his heart, protected from the chill of the winter of life, and the sound of his voice and the sense of his sheer strength bring comfort.[8]

The woman contains a bit of the man, and the man contains a bit of the woman; we each carry within us both masculine and feminine energies. However, as we reside in one dominant energy, we often lack a sense of peace regarding the polarities. For the Aquarian Sādhanā, Yogi Bhajan recommended that men recite one line and that women recite another of Jap Jī, and this is what we call a tantric-style recitation. Everyone recites the Mūl Mantra, or first stanza, together, then women recite the first line, which begins with "sochai soch," and the men follow with the second line, which begins with "chupai chup," and it alternates like this until the Salok at the end. Reciting this way assists us in harmonizing our feminine and masculine polarities: we don't have to like or even understand each other. The meditation recognizes our differences, honors them, and allows us to communicate with each other through the enlightening words of Jap Jī. We are healed in the process of listening and being listened to as we recite these sacred words.

"Jap Jī, Sukhmanī and Anand Sāhib are written
in Tantric Naad. These three Bānīs are in Tantric
Naad. You can read male and female lines and you
cannot believe how high you can become."

YOGI BHAJAN[9]

It's fine if you can't recite Jap Jī this way; just do the best you can with the voices of those present. I suggest, however, that you reserve the tantric-style recitation for when you have enough men and women to do it (even one of each works fine). However, if you are a group of women gathered together, I suggest you recite every single line together.

When I was sixteen, my older sister, Jiwan Shakti Kaur, took me to Goindwal, a holy well in India. It has eighty-four steps down a long tunnel to an underground well. As people have done for hundreds of years, you recite Jap Jī on each step followed by a dip in the well for each recitation. Slowly you descend, getting fully drenched in the well water and the vibration of Jap Jī with each step. My sister had done the practice quite a few times and was showing me the ropes. When we began on the highest and first step, I couldn't believe how fast she was reciting Jap Jī—something like eleven minutes per recitation! I tried to slow her down, but she just rolled her eyes. After about two steps, a half hour had passed, and I looked down and saw the remaining eighty-two steps yet to go; I suddenly realized the reason for her speed. We finished after eighteen hours, with only a couple of those hours spent for breaks. I can't describe how light, beautiful, and blessed I felt to have this experience with my sister. What an incredible feeling!

PRACTICAL APPLICATIONS OF JAP JĪ

Jap Jī is a tool meant to help us with daily life. Here are some practical applications:

- **Daily Recitation.** By beginning each day with these sound vibrations, we can intertwine the wisdom, love, and peace of the words into our being.

- **Birth and Death.** When we recite Jap Ji to a newborn, the sound current speaks to his or her subconscious and establishes the road map for the new soul to live in a divine way. We can also recite Jap Ji at the time of death. As the soul leaves the body, reciting Jap Ji can help it merge with the One.

- **Jap Ji as Prayer.** The vibration of Jap Ji can shift and change the energy of any situation to bring healing and transformation.

Here's an example of how I've used Jap Ji as prayer: One time on an airplane, I sat in an aisle seat as the rest of the passengers boarded. An elderly woman came down the aisle, appearing to be in a lot of pain as she winced with every step. A man—her husband, I assumed—followed her, a bit frazzled and carrying most of their luggage. When she stopped at my seat and saw me, the woman loudly protested, "Oh, no! We have to sit next to her?"

I quickly got up to let them in. The woman sat right next to me in the middle, her husband occupying the window seat and looking as if he wanted to jump out. The man gave me an apologetic look. Realizing that I couldn't make any small talk or that even a friendly smile might be rejected, I settled in for what appeared to be a long unpleasant five-hour experience. And as the engines began to rev up, so did this lady.

"I can't believe you didn't think of that!" she shouted at her husband, in one of her numerous rants and raves. "It's ridiculous. You never think of me! What a bozo you are!"

It kept going on and on for at least an hour. The husband shrank further down into his seat with each abuse thrown his way. I also began to feel more and more uncomfortable and uneasy. At some point, I realized I was beginning to feel as negative as the woman was acting. Funny how we can do that to each other as human beings.

Well, enough is enough, I thought. I pulled out my Jap Ji quietly, worried that she might see me and find something else to complain about. I began reciting it in a whisper, with the noise of the airplane humming right along. I chanted it from my heart and felt light coming from deep inside.

I wish I had some record of what happened next; if I could have filmed it, maybe you'd believe the incredible results. Within one minute of me reciting Jap Ji, the woman suddenly became quiet and peaceful, and she didn't rant for the rest of the trip! Thankfully, her husband was able to fall asleep. I owe this all (and so much more!) to Gurū Nānak. From the bottom of my heart, thank you!

It might not come in such a dramatic form, but I pray that Jap Ji will serve you in some way, no matter what your path may be. My friend, Ek Ong Kaar Kaur—a Jap Ji scholar—says it best: "Gurū Nānak held a truly Universal perspective; anyone, no matter what their faith, or spiritual inclination, will find something special for themselves in this beautiful song of soul known as Jap Ji."[10]

~ *Chapter Six* ~

BLISS IN THE BODY

Stage Three: Kundalini Yoga

ਭਾਠੀ ਗਗਨੁ ਸਿੰਙਿਆ ਅਰੁ ਚੁੰਙਿਆ ਕਨਕ ਕਲਸ ਇਕੁ ਪਾਇਆ ॥

bhāṭhī gagan sin(g)i-ā ar chun(g)i-ā kanak kalas ik pā-i-ā.

The Tenth Gate of my Crown Chakra is the distilling fire, and the Ida and Pingala are channels, to pour in and empty out the golden vat.

ਤਿਸੁ ਮਹਿ ਧਾਰ ਚੁਐ ਅਤਿ ਨਿਰਮਲ ਰਸ ਮਹਿ ਰਸਨ ਚੁਆਇਆ ॥੨॥

tis mah(i) dhār chu-ai at niramal ras mah(i) rasan chu-ā-i-ā. || 2 ||

Into that vat, there trickles a gentle stream of the most sublime and pure essence of all distilled essences.

ਏਕ ਜੁ ਬਾਤ ਅਨੂਪ ਬਨੀ ਹੈ ਪਵਨ ਪਿਆਲਾ ਸਾਜਿਆ ॥

ayk ju bāt anūp banī hai pavan pi-ālā sāji-ā.

Something wonderful has happened—the breath has become the cup.

ਤੀਨਿ ਭਵਨ ਮਹਿ ਏਕੋ ਜੋਗੀ ਕਹਹੁ ਕਵਨ ਹੈ ਰਾਜਾ ॥੩॥

tīn bhavan mah(i) ayko jogī kahah(u) kavan hai rājā. || 3||

In all the three worlds, such a Yogī is unique. What king can compare to him?

KABĪR JĪ, *SIRĪ GURŪ GRANTH SĀHIB JĪ*[1]

My husband first met Yogi Bhajan at Golden Bridge, the yoga center in Los Angeles where my husband began his practice. As it often is when spiritual masters come to visit, the whole center buzzed with excitment. People chatted away, staff members darted this way and that, and people kept streaming in the front door while he waited for Yogi Bhajan to come down the stairs.

And how he came down! Every time his left foot touched a step, he chanted "yo" and with his right foot, "ga." "Yo-ga, yo-ga, yo-ga, yo-ga!" All the way down the stairs.

Appropriately, Yogi Bhajan's class that night focused on the importance of yoga as a daily activity, especially since it's a step-by-step practice. With each repetition, we heal and release traumas and dramas and create space to experience our true essence. There is a miracle in every experience of yoga, but there are no overnight miracles. The yoking process takes time, as you might expect when considering that yoga is meant to unify body, mind, and soul.

Yogi Bhajan taught thousands of classes; thankfully, a large number of these were recorded. Of all the wonderful yoga sets he offered, I'm only including a few of my favorites here. Yogi Bhajan received these sets from the Golden Chain I talked about in chapter 3, so whenever we engage in a Kundalini Yoga set, we experience the mastery and lineage of the entire Golden Chain, of which Yogi Bhajan is but one link. The Golden Chain is present in every Kundalini Yoga experience—guiding, protecting, and healing. For this reason, we practice the sets exactly as taught, without mixing in other techniques.

In appendix B you will find nine Kundalini Yoga sets, or Kriyas, outlined in detail with model images for you to follow along with. I specifically chose these Kriyas because I found they work quite well in the morning; I love all of them, and I've included a range for people with different physical abilities. Please keep in mind that you can enjoy these sets at any time of the day (although the Kriya for Morning Sādhanā is best in the morning). I advise picking one set and doing it every day until you become very familiar with it. In fact, a minimum of a forty-day practice, as I will discuss later, is highly recommended. Please continue reading to become familiar with the energetics of each set, and choose one based on what you are attracted to and what you feel you need. Intuition is key here, so perhaps you can take a moment or many moments to close your eyes and take a few deep breaths as you decide. You could also work with a certified Kundalini Yoga instructor (information is listed in the resources section) to help you determine where to begin.

My husband is a wonderul yogī and incredible Kundalini Yoga teacher. Often when we teach workshops together, I teach the chanting and he teaches the yoga. We thoroughly discussed the yoga sets detailed in this book, and we want to offer our personal experience with each to support you in the journey as you become familiar with them. I don't expect that you'll have an experience identical to my own—that's part of the magic of Kundalini Yoga.

SŪRYA NAMASKĀRA — SUN SALUTATIONS

Yogi Bhajan suggested Sun Salutations as an excellent warm-up before any Kundalini Yoga Kriya, or practice. Specifically, he noted that Sun Salutations increase circulation, stretch the spine, massage the organs, aid in digestion, and oxygenate the blood. I recommend doing at least three rounds and increasing to five or six. Sun Salutations create space in the body; this helps clear out emotional energy, but it also makes room for positive energy to flow. The amount of positivity can be overwhelming! As we create space for this new influx, we can carry it in a balanced way and bring the energy into our lives with intelligence and ease.

BASIC SPINAL ENERGY SERIES

As it says in the instructor's manual for this practice: "Age is measured by the flexibility of the spine; to stay young, stay flexible. This series works systematically from the base of the spine to the top. All twenty-six vertebrae receive stimulation, and all the Chakras receive a burst of energy. This makes it a good series to do before meditation. Many people report greater mental clarity after regular practice of this Kriya. A contributing factor is the increased circulation of the spinal fluid, which is crucially linked to having a good memory."[2]

This set is ideal for someone just starting out with yoga or someone who lacks flexibility. It works with the energy of the spine—a key place to start increasing our flexibility throughout the body. After practicing it one morning, I was surprised to find that I was much more flexible in my legs and arms than before. If you can't sit on the floor, feel free to do this set in a chair, and please review the instructions in appendix B for more specifics.

Although many people consider this set "easy" physically, I have been astounded by the depth of my own experience with it, and I've grown to respect its power and beauty. I get a deep sense of positive well-being, balance, and spacious perspective on life when I do this set, and this is precisely the zenith of the Kundalini experience.

Pay special attention to the rests specified in between the exercises in this set. We tend to overlook the rests and just go from movement to movement, as this is our normal operating procedure. Practice this set and take the rests as instructed: it will really help to move energy up your spine. You might find the relaxation at the end challenging, but remember how important it is to have this space for yourself.

The Bear Grip portion of this set (holding the breath in and out) can bring up painful memories and sensations. If this happens, please notice the hurt, hold yourself with love, and make space for the experience; this is how we can finally release the pain. The last exercise before the relaxation is Sat Kriya, one of the most important Kriyas in Kundalini Yoga. It heals any imbalances in the lower triangle (the first three Chakras), thereby allowing us to move up to our higher center of being at the fourth Chakra, the Heart Center.

AWAKENING TO YOUR TEN BODIES

This is the first sequence I memorized as a teenager and remains the one I come back to most often in my daily practice. It has brought me much joy and peace in my life. I love especially how it stretches and moves different areas of the body, including an incredible series of exercises that open up the spine.

What differentiates this set from other Kriyas in Kundalini Yoga is that in the beginning you focus on the navel intensely with Stretch Pose.

This key exercise can totally set your navel center in place, grounding you to live in your strength regardless of what you face in life. In the context of this Kriya, Stretch Pose grounds you in your physical body, which is essential in order to awaken the other facets of the self.

At the conclusion of this set, you'll find the chanting practice called Laya Yoga Meditation. As teenagers we loved to really belt this one out. I encourage you to do the same! Maybe you'll also experience the delightful sensation of the Kundalini energy rising.

KRIYA FOR ELEVATION

This simple Kriya touches upon key areas in our body that allow for a sensation of elevation. It works with the energy of Prāna, and as that energy moves up the spine, we receive the opportunity to release, let go, and heal. Tension, bad habits, worries, and fears energetically live in the body in certain locations. In the same way that washing our car clears off mud spots and dusting reveals a shiny exterior, our practice brings a new sensation of awakening that feels incredibly refreshing after existing for so long in a state of confusion and distrust. We realize that we don't need those bad habits any longer, and we don't even want them. We fall in love with the experience of awakening, serenity, and peace; we start to want it. In this set, it all comes from the spine. As we practice the Sat Kriya at the end, we totally elevate and tap into this new reality—who we are and who we have always been.

KRIYA FOR MORNING SĀDHANĀ

Yogi Bhajan originally taught this set in Morning Sādhanā in 1971, before I was born, but I can easily visualize him teaching it in that loving way he had. This set touches different areas of the body, so it's a delightful set for the morning when you want to send Prāna throughout your body. There are several exercises, but none of them take very long to do. I suggest you move right through them without breaks in between unless specified.

One of the greatest gifts of this set happens at the end of the last exercise, where you are asked to sit and meditate for one minute. All of the preceding movement (especially the second-to-last exercise) primes you for a deep meditative experience. Although it's short, my husband notes how beneficial even one minute can be. He says, "You get this minute where you are just sitting there, and you are amazed by how still, silent, and peaceful it feels inside. Even just that one minute is a gift. It sets you for the day. In that one minute, it is like you just brought your car to the best mechanic in the world, he totally tuned it up and fixed it up, and you are ready to go for another three thousand miles. You know there will be potholes, times when you will have to hit the brakes, and times when you will have to accelerate to get on the freeway. But you brought it into the shop, and it is ready. After that one minute, you are set with practice for the next twenty-four hours. And it is not like you need more, really; that experience of stillness stays with you. It is for your well-being, balance, and joy."

MAGNETIC FIELD AND HEART CENTER

This set works to strengthen the magnetic field and heart center. We create the magnetic field—the energy space around us—with our internal vibration, and it communicates and relates to our surroundings.

You will find in this set quite a bit of engagement of the navel center, an area that many experience as energetically dense. However, when we move this part of our body physically or etherically with Prāna, two things can happen: a deep sense of belonging in our body and a clearing of the pathway that connects the navel center to the heart center. With the strength of the navel engaged, we feel safe, and we experience the compassion of an open heart.

Keeping an open heart is a continuous process. You can't keep an open heart by engaging in a set once; you have to do it repeatedly. Over time, resistance and residue of emotional energy builds inside, and you have to clean it out and let it go. You might find challenging moments in this set that provide you an opportunity to meet physical and mental limits; these will help you discover expansion within yourself and assist you in experiencing the magnetic field. When you create the space in the center of your being that is whole, open, thriving, and at peace, that energy radiates out into your magnetic field, and this directly affects how people experience you. We're all connected. As your magnetic field communicates messages of well-being to others, those people are brought into their own sense of okayness, either consciously or unconsciously. Additionally, we become better able to pass through challenging situations arising from ourselves or the environment, and we emerge on the other side of difficulties with our hearts open and willing to share this openness with others.

I encourage you to truly listen to your own voice in the two wonderful chants in this set, and if you are practicing with others, please take the opportunity to listen to their voices as well. Listening is essential in order to heal ourselves and each other.

PITUITARY GLAND SERIES

The pituitary gland sits at the center of the skull, behind the eyes, where the optic nerves cross over behind the bridge of the nose. By supporting the pituitary in this practice, we rejuvenate the entire body through the neuroendocrine link. This set creates a particular kind of opening in our physical body: as the pituitary gland is supported and stimulated, we feel it radiating out to our entire body, all the way to our toes and fingertips. Through the beautiful elongating movements of this set, we create a spaciousness within our physical body so that our spirit and our breath have room to be. We feel light and clear for the rest of the day.

When we support the pituitary gland, we manifest the subtle energy qualities of the sixth Chakra, one of which is intuition. The stronger our intuition, the more capable we become of making choices that support the unfolding of our destiny, and this harmonizes us with the love of the cosmos and the universal flow that exists within everyone. In this way, what is good for the individual is good for all. Intuition acts as a source of light that we can tap into every day; it shows us the way and tunes us in to the reality of truth. Accordingly, we meet challenges with a lightness of being because part of us already knows how things will unfold.

STRESS SET FOR ADRENALS AND KIDNEYS

When we become overly stressed, our adrenals and kidneys need extra support. Biologically and energetically, this set really helps with that, as I can personally attest. After practicing this set, I feel much lighter and more relaxed—truly welcome experiences when I've been stressed! Our organs benefit from genuine relaxation, which enables them to rest and heal. The relaxation period in this set lasts a full hour, and I recommend doing it for the entire hour, if possible; it may make up your entire morning practice, but it is well worth it if you are currently struggling with stress. You can also perform this set with the full relaxation period at other times of day that may work for you (just before bed, for example). And if you don't have a full hour to devote to the relaxation, I recommend incorporating at least an eleven-minute relaxation.

The sensation of stress can feel quite lonely, but we aren't truly alone. The yogīs who developed and practiced this set knew all about stress and how to deal with it, so they passed this technology down to us. Just keeping that in mind helps me feel less lonely. Far back into the past, human beings lived and toiled and worried just like us; better yet, they discovered ways to make this life more manageable. So let us relax, do our best, and keep smiling.

As my Kundalini Yoga teacher and mentor, Hari Kirin Kaur Khalsa, says, this set offers particular benefits to women: "The Stress Set for the Adrenals and Kidneys is wonderful for anyone experiencing stress but is especially helpful for women in perimenopause and menopause. During perimenopause, when our ovaries decrease production of estrogen and progesterone, our adrenals are called on to make smaller amounts of these hormones. They also regulate minerals in the body, aid in digestion, and work with the thyroid to maintain energy levels. If the adrenals are already stressed when you enter perimenopause and menopause, it is more difficult for them to assume these new tasks."[3]

YOGA FOR MENSTRUAL HEALTH AND RELIEF

I feel so grateful to have a husband who acknowledges my need for space during my menstrual cycle. This time is incredibly important for the soul of a woman, and to be able to meditate during the cycle offers tremendous benefits. For countless generations, women of the First Nations (indigenous people of Canada) had lodges to experience their Moon Time alone. They viewed this period as a time when the veils between the physical and spirit worlds were at their thinnest, and therefore a woman could access deep states of meditation to gain tools and strength to reenter the community and daily life. So I encourage you to find a way to spend time alone for at least some of your Moon Time. For me, the best kind of alone time includes meditation. As I mentioned before, when following the practices I've outlined, don't take a cold shower during your Moon Time; use warm water, and enjoy a bath if possible! Take it easy. Drink warm tea. I've included some supporting exercises for you here, as well; some to help with overall menstrual health that you can practice any time, and others that are specifically beneficial for relieving menstrual cramping.

KUNDALINI YOGA GUIDELINES

I attended a friend's office-warming party. She's a Kundalini Yoga teacher who was kicking off her career as an acupuncturist.

"You see that man over there?" she asked. An elderly man sat in a chair, laughing and talking with the woman next to him. His light blue eyes twinkled with joy.

"He started coming to my class a few months ago. He'd never done Kundalini Yoga before—he totally loved it and signed up for every class in town he could find. He was in a walker when he first started, and now he doesn't need to use his walker any more. Pretty cool, eh?"

Pretty cool indeed. You might not experience such dramatic benefits, but I guarantee this practice will help you in some way. So, let's get down to basics.

Beginning Your Practice

At the beginning of every Kundalini Yoga class, as well as the start of the Aquarian Sādhanā, we tune in with the Ādī Mantra before we begin. Tuning in with this Mantra aligns us with the Golden

Chain—Yogi Bhajan, Gurū Rām Dās, and all who hold these teachings sacred. As Yogi Bhajan said, when we chant this Mantra, we "manifest Infinity through the Grace of Gurū Rām Dās."[4] As we tune in, our ego—whether we're teacher or student—steps aside so that the purity of the teachings may come through. This Mantra acts as a call to the Divine that we may awaken and be brought to the original light of the soul within.

We chant the Ādī Mantra three times, following these repetitions with the Mangala Charan Mantra, which we also chant three to five times. This second Mantra, although optional, surrounds our practice with a protective energy.

ĀDĪ MANTRA

ong namo

I bow to the energy of the Divine within myself and all beings

gurū dayv namo

I bow to the Divine teacher within myself and within all beings

MANGALA CHARAN MANTRA

ādguray namah

I bow to the primal Gurū, that which takes us from darkness to light

jugād guray namah

I bow to the Gurū throughout the ages

satiguray namah

I bow to the True Gurū

sirī gurdayvay namah

I bow to the Great Divine Gurū

Posture

Sit in a comfortable cross-legged position with a straight spine. Place the palms of your hands together as if in prayer, with fingers pointing straight up, and then press the joints of the thumbs into the center of your chest. Inhale deeply. Focus on your Third Eye Point. As you exhale, chant the entire Ādī Mantra in one breath. After doing this three times, follow with three repetitions of the Mangala Charan Mantra.[5]

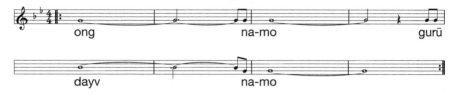

Musical Notation for Tuning In with the Ādī Mantra

Timing

All of the yoga sets (or Kriyas) given by Yogi Bhajan work scientifically; they are absolutely precise and effective. He knew from his own personal mastery exactly how long each Kriya would take to do its work. If you can do the time amounts as given in the manual for each exercise, that's wonderful, but please do not exceed the time. If you can't practice the Kriyas as they were given, you can proportionately cut each exercise down. The important thing is to keep the ratios the same within all of the exercises because the whole set works on you in a beautiful orchestration of chemical reactions and soul awakenings. For example, if you only have twenty minutes for a set that would take forty in its suggested length, reduce the time you spend on each exercise by half.

If you need to take breaks while performing an exercise, that's entirely fine. However, please keep your breaks within reason and maintain your intention to complete the exercise in its full prescribed time at some point. Respect your body's limitations and keep in mind that it may take some time to build up your stamina and strength. Often people who begin practicing Kundalini Yoga are not just learning to do specific yoga sets; they are also shifting to a healthier diet and lifestyle. It may take time to flush the body of toxins and be able to perform a Kundalini Yoga set as specified.

Mixing and Matching

We do not combine other forms of yoga with a Kundalini Yoga set. Because these sets work with sensitive and subtle systems of the body, keeping the integrity of the set as given is extremely important. If you have other techniques you would like to add that work for you, please do! But make sure you complete the Kundalini Yoga set before you move on to other techniques.

Leading Versus Teaching

There are some notable differences between leading Sādhanā and teaching a yoga class. For the Aquarian Sādhanā, you do not need to be a certified Kundalini Yoga teacher to lead the morning yoga practice. However, keep in mind the following if you plan on leading a group Sādhanā in your community:

Although you may have experienced music in a Kundalini Yoga class before, we tend to keep it quiet during the Amrit Vaylā, without any music for the morning yoga unless specified in the original teachings of Yogi Bhajan. We also advise that you not talk a lot. You can give the basic instructions or clarifications as needed, but please minimize the talking. In other settings, a Kundalini Yoga teacher may employ lots of inspirational stories or other tools to help and encourage, but we keep the feeling quiet and serene in the morning so that people have the opportunity to practice and become aware of their internal and external experience with as little verbal input from the leader as possible.

If you wish to lead a particular set, practice it ahead of time until you reach a state of comfort with it. Read the instructions carefully, too, and do so each time! It is easy to forget or "change" something in the set inadvertently. When you lead the yoga set during the Aquarian Sādhanā, you can practice right along with everyone. If you become a Kundalini Yoga teacher, you will most likely sit and support people with your meditative presence as opposed to performing sets along with them. But in Sādhanā, you can simply practice along with everyone else.

Note to Women

As I mentioned before, I've included two series of exercises to help you during your menstrual cycle: you can practice the first every day as a way to improve how you feel when your cycle comes; the second series can help relieve menstrual cramping. During the heavy part of your menstruation, stay away from Breath of Fire (which is described below) or postures that invert your uterus, and please decide on your own when it feels good to resume these positions. During menstruation, our energy moves downward as we go through this important cleansing time, so we support this process with our yoga as well.

If you are pregnant, doing a morning practice is the best thing you can do for yourself. Check out the prenatal resources listed at the end of this book. There are wonderful DVDs and manuals specializing in Kundalini Yoga instruction for pregnant women, and I highly recommend them. We are blessed with so many incredible teachings!

Relaxation

An incredible amount of work happens in our nervous, endocrine, circulatory, and muscular systems while we engage in Kundalini Yoga exercises. There is often a Deep Relaxation at the end of each set that is important for integrating all of the healing benefits into the systems of our bodies. However, the relaxations in between each posture while you are practicing the set are just as important. Unless the manual specifies to move directly into the next exercise, take a few moments to allow the energy of the exercise to resonate within you and settle in a bit before moving on.

For Deep Relaxation, allow your body to rest lying on your back. Be sure to rest with the full weight of your legs on the floor. Sometimes people relax with their knees up in the air, but this takes energy from your body, as your muscles must work to keep your legs up. Try to relax without any pillows or props; the weight of your natural body will do wonders for you. Allow the palms to face up at your sides, and cover yourself with a shawl or blanket to keep cozy and warm. This is a perfect opportunity to just let go and feel the Creator holding you. How wonderful to know that you are taken care of! Feel it, allow it, and relax. As the Aquarian teacher instructor manual says, "Deep relaxation allows you to enjoy and consciously integrate the mind-body changes which have been brought about during the practice of this Kriya. It allows you to sense the extension of the self through the magnetic field and the Aura and allows the physical body to deeply relax."[6] How wonderful!

After your Deep Relaxation, practice the following set of exercises.[7]

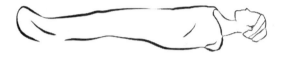

Deep Relaxation

COMING OUT OF DEEP RELAXATION EXERCISES

Gently come back into your body awareness, or invite others to do so if you are leading. A good way to do this is to take a long, deep breath.

1. Rotate your wrists and ankles in both directions. Then rub the palms of your hands and the soles of your feet together.

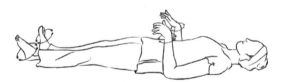

Rotate Wrists and Ankles

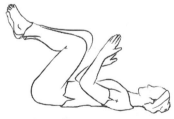

Rub Palms and Soles of Feet

2. With your arms stretched out to either side, bring the right knee over to the left side of the body to touch the floor, and look to your right in what is called Cat Stretch. Switch sides a few times.

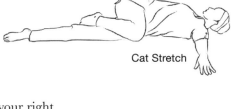

Cat Stretch

3. Rock back and forth a few times on your back.

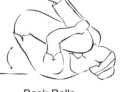

Back Rolls

ENDING YOUR PRACTICE

If you are only doing a Kundalini Yoga set for your morning practice, please finish with the song called "Long Time Sun." You can find it in chapter 8.

KUNDALINI YOGA TERMS

A man came up to me after a concert in Montreal. He said that a couple of weeks before he had a dream in which the word *Kundalini* came to him. The sound of the word resounded in his dream so much that when he awoke the next morning it was all he could think of. *Kundalini, Kundalini, Kundalini . . .*

He had no idea what the word meant. He said, "I thought it was a kind of pasta!"

A few days later he saw a flier advertising an evening of chanting with me, including "chants from the Kundalini Yoga tradition." The flier steered him to our concert. He reported loving the experience, and it encouraged him to begin his journey with Kundalini Yoga at the local yoga center.

By now you know that Kundalini doesn't refer to some kind of pasta, but to clarify other important words, I'll review some key terms below.

Bandhas

Kundalini Yoga frequently employs locks (Bandhas). These combinations of muscle contractions improve nerve function, circulation, and the flow of cerebral spinal fluid, in addition to directing Prāna in such a way as to raise the Kundalini energy. Bandhas further focus energy for self-healing. The most important locks are Jalandhar Bandh, Uddiyana Bandh, and Mūlbandh. Jalandhar Bandh, or Neck Lock, is one of the most highly used locks. Gently elongate the back of the neck, and slightly tuck the chin in. Elevate the chest slightly, making sure to relax the face and neck muscles. This creates a straight line from the base of the spine to the top of the head and draws your energy upward. Uddiyana Bandh, or Diaphragm Lock, is practiced only on the exhale. With the spine straight, this lock is applied by lifting the diaphragm up high into the thorax and pulling the upper abdominal muscles back toward the spine. As senior Kundalini Yoga teacher Gurucharan Singh says, "Uddiyana Bandh gently massages the intestines and the heart muscle."[8] Mūlbandh Bandh, or Root Lock, is a powerful and potent lock. *Mūl* means the root, and this lock concentrates our Prāna at the root of our being where the Kundalini energy can rise. To begin, pull in the rectum, then the sex organ so that the urethral tract is contracted, then pull in the navel center. Once you are comfortable with these three movements in that sequence, you can then move to the next level and pull in all three at the same time.

Breath of Fire

Kundalini Yoga Kriyas often include this technique; it takes time to get comfortable with its rapid, rhythmic, and continuous pace. The breath is equally long on the inhalation and exhalation, with no pause between, at approximately two to three breaths per second. Breath of Fire comes through the nose, mouth closed—a relaxed, balanced contraction and relaxation of the diaphragm. When exhaling, the navel moves back toward the spine; inhaling just happens as the navel relaxes. The chest stays slightly lifted throughout the breathing cycle. Gurucharan Singh states, "Breath of Fire is a cleansing breath, renewing the blood and releasing old toxins from the lungs, mucus linings, blood vessels, and cells. It is a powerful way to adjust your autonomic nervous system and get rid of stress."[9] If you practice it regularly, your lungs soon increase their capacity to expand, and you will not only be able to increase your pace but it also becomes a very enjoyable breath.

Original Sparkle

If we could only preserve the sparkle in a laughing child's eyes! If only we could keep that sparkle in a special box in order to peek in from time to time so we could feel the pure joy that opened our hearts. The experience of Kundalini Yoga resembles this sparkle. It's not something that one can explain very well with words or pictures (as I'm trying to do here!), but I've no doubt that you can feel it lighting and warming your heart. I pray that you will, by the Grace of the Love of the Universe, experience that original sparkle.

~ *Chapter Seven* ~

CHANTING AS THE SUN RISES

Stage Four: Aquarian Sādhanā Mantras

ਹਰਿ ਹਰਿ ਨਾਮੁ ਨਿਧਾਨੁ ਹੈ ਗੁਰਮੁਖਿ ਪਾਇਆ ਜਾਇ ॥

har har nām nidhān hai guramukh pā-i-ā jā-i.

The Name of the Lord, Har, Har, is the greatest bliss.
The Gurmukhs (those attuned to the Gurū) obtain it.

GURŪ RĀM DĀS, *SIRĪ GURŪ GRANTH SĀHIB JĪ*[1]

The sweetness of the Aquarian Sādhanā lies in the experience of chanting. As a musician, I will admit to being biased. My mother tells me that as a young child I would sleep through the whole Sādhanā, but when the chanting started I would often pop up and join in. Now as an adult, I dearly love every aspect of this practice, but I have journeyed most deeply into the chanting.

Taking a cold shower and doing yoga primes you for a blissful chanting experience. I think there is almost no way your Kundalini energy won't rise! If you have come this far and chant these words, the energy of your Chakra system and all of your ten bodies will be present and engaged. For this stage, just enjoy, enjoy, enjoy! The music and the energy of the chants will take you out of your everyday mind—this is the merger of the Lover and the Beloved. It's your time with God. The energetics of each chant,

97

the order, and timing create a healing sonic formula. One goes through a journey of self-awakening and discovery from the start of the chants to the end. For this reason I highly encourage you to practice the chants in the order and with the specific times as listed in appendix C as they are each an important element in a very purposeful healing experience. If this feels daunting to you, please do what you can, and you can see "Ideas to Begin Your Journey" in chapter 9 for ways to start.

Yogi Bhajan encouraged the musicians in our community to bring their music to the practices of Kundalini Yoga, including the Aquarian Sādhanā. As we learned the traditional Sikh style of music from which the chants come, we included touches of classical music, folk, jazz, and rock 'n' roll. As long as these elements supported the Naad, or sacred sound current, Yogi Bhajan loved and honored the innovations. Music is indeed an incredible gift. You may experience, as I often do, the hypnotic quality that supportive music brings to meditation. When the chanting starts, music helps me lose my thoughts and merge into a place of loving meditation with the One. That's why I included the *Light of the Naam with Long Ek Ong Kar* CD to support your practice, and I encourage you to use it as long as it works for you. I also welcome you to find other artists in this community who have recorded wonderful Sādhanā CDs or even to create music of your own!

Following are some other ways to support your practice.

HOW TO SET YOURSELF

Prepare to sit for the duration of the chants, making sure to hydrate and empty your bladder if needed. Cover yourself with something warm and make sure you sit on something comfortable that supports your hips. Sit in Easy Pose, a seated, cross-legged position that encourages a straight spine and allows one to experience meditative ease and stillness. Pull in the chin slightly with Neck Lock (page 94) to establish a straight line from the base of the spine to the

Easy Pose

top of the head. Bring the tip of your Jupiter, or index finger, to the tip of your thumb in Giān Mudra; this opens the door to the energy of Jupiter, which represents expansion and journeying beyond the known into the unknown. Once you have learned the Mantras, closing your eyes will help turn your energies inward. Focus the eyes at the Third Eye Point to further quiet the mind. It is especially important to cover your spine and head for this practice; it encourages the Kundalini energy to rise and creates stability within. This is the posture that was given to us for the first chant of the morning called "Long Ek Ong Kār." Most mornings I stay in this posture for all of the chants, save one chant that has a specific posture, "Wāhegurū Wāhe Jī-o." I will go into more detail with that a little later in this chapter.

CHANTING WITH BREATH

Yogic chanting is a particularly conscious form of breathing, or *Prānayam*. After chanting we feel uplifted because we literally *lift up* our energy. Experiencing this, however, means that a lot of factors must line up: the Grace of the Divine, the Grace of the Gurū, the Mercy of the Beloved, and—most within our control—the degree to which we apply ourselves to the breath and to our chanting. In order to fully experience the uplifting energy of the Mantra, we must fully engage our breath and align with the sacred sounds. When I compose tunes for any kind of chanting, I try to remain acutely aware of the breath. Between recitations, we fill our lungs, and that drops us fully into our being. It is through the breath that we live! So to really enjoy the chanting experience, I encourage you to take full, deep breaths as you chant. Then you can truly hear your voice and fall in love with it. When your own voice embodies words of inspiration, words of the Divine, it becomes the agent that reveals and transforms you into the beautiful being that you are.

WHEN THOUGHTS ARISE

Don't worry about thoughts coming up as you chant; it's natural. Chanting cleans and clears our subconscious, and the Mantra creates a vortex that pulls out the energy of the subconscious that is no longer useful. It pulls out grief; it pulls out despair; it pulls out anger. Some of this process you will be aware of in your conscious mind, but most you won't actually perceive—the only indication will be a torrent of thoughts, all meant on some level to keep the deep work of clearing the subconcious from happening. Why? Because we get comfortable in habitual energy patterns; without them, we must do the work to change. Even worse, we come to realize that we have to give up the illusion of control. Try something different here: instead of taking the various bait dangled by the scared aspects of your mind—brilliant ideas for work, ways to improve your parenting, what you should have said to your rude neighbor—just notice the thought and return to the Mantra. This simple redirection of your attention will take you to the inner silence. Call it forth. Sink deeper, beyond the thoughts. That's where you'll find the true food and nourishment of your practice.

CHANTING IN A GROUP

We have talked a lot about the internal experience. Now let's take it deeper; let's talk about group Sādhanā. To begin with, Yogi Bhajan taught us to sing in unison, to sing as one being, so try that with your own group.[2] Try to merge with your environment; in group Sādhanā, this means your neighbors. Sometimes people sing too loudly, sometimes too quietly, and sometimes out of tune. That happens, of course, but I encourage you and the members of your group to focus on supporting the group as a whole. It doesn't particularly matter what musical gifts you do or don't have; what matters is that the whole group sings together to bring forth a wonderful golden energy. When you accomplish this, you may discover that there is nothing more powerful on this planet. I remember Yogi Bhajan often saying, "To understand is to stand under." Understand each other, serve each other, and love each other.

FEELING TIRED?

Some people go to sleep during the chants. That's okay, too. Sometimes when you practice Sādhanā, you'll be tired or sick, and when you sit down, the need for extra rest will show itself. Keep in mind that just sitting with the vibrations will promote healing. However, if you regularly find yourself becoming sleepy during chanting, you need to take a look at how much sleep you're getting, what you're eating and drinking, and any other factors regarding your physical health. This will help you determine what you need to do to remain alert for the experience.

A NOTE TO MUSICIANS

When I compose tunes for any kind of chanting, I make sure that I can sing each syllable clearly and with enough breath—there should be plenty of space to breathe. I also pay attention to the pace of the chants because going too fast shortens the breath and compromises pronunciation, and both of these weaken the effect of the Mantra. As well, going too slowly diminishes the fire or warmth of the chanting experience, and unless you find yourself playing music for incredibly deep meditators, you may in fact put people to sleep!

I also pay attention to the pitch. After spending a lot of time with people in chanting situations, I have come to understand the vocal range that most people feel comfortable with. And especially in the early morning hours, it's lower than you would expect. It starts off at a low A and moves up about five to eight notes from there, and more often than not, it stays in the lower range of those notes.

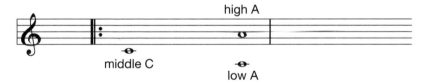

Recommended Note Range for Morning Chanting

As a musician, you want your music to help people chant. The more people experience the energy of the chants, the more they will heal. The stimulation of the hypothalamus, through the tapping of the tongue on the roof of the mouth, results in a complete orchestration of the Kundalini rising, in which messages of health and well-being course through the entire body. Remember this process as you compose.

When someone chants the Aquarian Sādhanā with you, let them do it in such a way that they can sit in stillness and royalty.

Keep the tunes simple and repetitive to foster a state of deep meditation. By suddenly inserting a bridge, changing keys, or including an instrumental, we break the trance, and that trance is ever so important in someone's journey inward. If, after Sādhanā, people remember what an incredible musician you are, or how great you played, then you have failed in your job. Instead, let your music take them deep within to remember who they are, assisting them to connect with the Mantra; this will lighten their spirits so that they may soar throughout the rest of the day with every breath they take.

I love harmonies, but I try to use them sparingly. Harmonies add a little glory and gold to the chanting, but keep them subtle so they don't take over the experience in any way. Remember, all aspects of your music should support the group voice as it develops throughout the morning. Harmonies can confuse some participants as they try to figure out whether to sing the lead vocal or the harmony. People who have mastered the art of chanting do not typically perform on stage—they live in small villages in India, gather in Gurdwārās and temples, play whatever instruments they can get their hands on, and sit on dirt floors. However, they sing together in unison, with humility and joy. Remember this. Keep it simple. And you too will find that door to salvation.

As musicians, we engage with the energy that lives within and around us. We work against this energy when we try to perform or impress. When we engage this energy, however, we become deeply present and find the key to our hearts—we find God. Everything becomes a conversation with the Divine—the sound of raindrops falling, the welcome smell of a meditation space, the psychic vibration of those attending Sādhanā, and our own internal vibration. We are all works in progress as we complete our karmas, learn the lessons needed to move forward in life, and find the truth within us. Really feel the environment—the air, the people, the music—and sing to all of that. Allow the Mantra to heal. If you do this, people will experience you singing to their soul. What more could you ask for?

As musicians we serve the meditative experience. Can we serve the experience and be fully in it at the same time? The answer is both no and yes. No, because you will not experience the same kind of Kundalini rising felt when one sits still. But you will experience something even greater: the positive energy that comes from serving others in delivering this uplifting experience.

Lastly, because we musicians have the capacity to transfer healing to others, we must remain healthy ourselves in body, mind, and spirit. The Aquarian Sādhanā is a wonderful practice for musicians. Every day, we have the opportunity to tap into our craft, to discipline ourselves, and to practice merging with the Mantra. In addition to generating positive health and stability, the Sādhanā also has the power to enrich our musical life.

LIVE MUSIC AND COMMUNITY BUILDING

I hope you like the recorded music included with this manual. I also recommend using versions of the Aquarian Sādhanā available from other talented artists. However, the best results come from experiencing live music. Music heals. It nurtures communities and helps them grow. I liken it to making a good batch of yogurt: First you heat the milk until it boils—that's the Jap Jī recitation and yoga. Then you stir in two tablespoons of prepared yogurt and put it in an oven on low heat—that's the chanting with live music. After letting it sit in that vibration for the right amount of time, you get a wonderful batch of yogurt, and from that batch, you take two tablespoons and create the next batch of yogurt. In this way, you are set for life. Every batch of yogurt just gets better and better. And so it is with live music and the community. You create a culture of love, light, and joy that grows, that vibrates, that serves, without words and without ego, through the gifts and talents and spiritual devotion of its own people. That culture creates graceful, beautiful, secure, and loving environments for your community.

Any community that supports live Sādhanā every day will greatly benefit. As musicians, when we provide live music in this way, we reach out to the energy within and around us, and we merge with it. As the participants meditate, we musicians go deeper, and as we go deeper, we guide others to do the same. This results in a truly beautiful dance of blessed, exciting, and living energy. I find that live music, experienced as either the musician or the listener, makes it easier to enter a state of thoughtlessness and depth in meditation. I encourage you to create a community of musicians who support each other and take turns leading. A healthy culture requires variety and consistency; it requires something living and real. Find it, and victory will be yours.

EFFECTS AND MEANING OF EACH CHANT

In this section we go into the mantras and their meanings. For your daily practice, please find a more succinct listing of the Mantras in appendix C.

The language of these chants, for the most part, comes from Gurmukhī, so the words are meant to impart healing and consciousness. Each word contributes to this experience, whether we know the meaning or not. These chants are poems—expressive, sacred songs. They offer rich connotations, vivid descriptions, and lively metaphors for life. So to more fully understand the art form and experience its impact, let's look at the meaning of each word—a practice my mother, Prabhu Nam Kaur, taught me. I feel so grateful to her for guiding me through this process and helping me with the meanings of many of these words. I encourage you to contemplate each word in a relaxed space and get to know the meanings little by little; even a little understanding will support your meditation. We'll explore each of them here.

THE ĀDĪ SHAKTĪ: LONG EK ONG KĀR

ek ong kār, sat nām sirī, wāhegurū.

The Creator and all Creation are one, this is our true identity, the ecstasy of wisdom is great beyond words.[3]

- ek: the one vibration within all of us

- ong: manifested vibration of the Divine; the sound current from which all Creation arises

- kār: to do, to make; that which does, makes, or creates

- sat: the vibration of truth

- nām: identity; the Name of God that vibrates through all beings and is what creates us; the creative vibration that is within; I am, I am

- sirī: great; God is great

- wāhegurū: ecstatic is the experience of the Gurū, the One who takes us from darkness to light

This first Mantra vibrates up the entire spine, from the base to the top of the head. Practicing it helps us initiate, experience, and celebrate the Divine resonance of Kundalini energy within us. I first connected with this Mantra as a teenager at yoga camp in the scenic mountains of Arizona. Every morning before sunrise, the head of the camp would get up, climb to the top of the roof of our cabin, and chant this Mantra at the top of his lungs for two and a half hours. Soon the sun would sparkle golden and silver through his greying beard, each note punctuated by the movement of his navel in passionate strokes. He was so purely connected with God through this practice, and everyone felt it. He never tried to inspire or directly ask any of us to join him, but we did happily, like bees drawn to the scent of a sacred flower. We chanted along with him, dropping into an inner space of love that I would never forget. As the sun rose higher into the sky, I remember feeling abundant, full, and totally content in my heart, having everything my soul ever wanted in those rich moments of union with the Divine.

The Long Ek Ong Kār Mantra is done with a two-and-a-half-breath cycle. You take one long deep breath and chant "ek ong kār," inhale again and chant "sat nām, sirī," then take a half breath and chant "wāhegurū." We don't use musical accompaniment here, although what happens inside the body is a total orchestral celebration as this Mantra vibrates through the spine, stimulates the Chakra system, and awakens the Kundalini.

For the whole recitation, apply the Root Lock (or Mūlbandh), pulling in the rectum, genitals, and navel center up and in toward the spine. You can also engage Neck Lock (Jalandhar Bandh), with your chin slightly tucked in, creating a straight line from the base of the spine to the top of the head. (Please refer to the "Bandhas" section in chapter 6 for more information on the locks.) Now as you chant "ek," pull up on the navel center. As you chant "ong," like with the conch shell, allow the sound to resonate in your skull and the base of your nose. With "kār," the sound resonates out from the navel and heart center, generating an open feeling. Inhale deeply, then on "sat" pull in the navel again, and expand on "nām," using up most of the breath. At the end of the breath, chant "sirī" and pull in the Uddiyana Bandh, or Diaphragm Lock. With "sirī," pause as you pull the diaphragm in. Inhale briefly and pull in your navel to send out the short, powerful sound of "wāh," softening into completion with "he-gurū." Each time you pull the navel at "ek," "sat," and "wāh," also make that a time to strengthen your Mūlbandh, pulling in on the rectum, genitals, and navel. After chanting "gurū," consciously pull in the Mūlbandh at the very end to concentrate the energy and prepare to begin the cycle of the Mantra again. As stated before, here is the posture and eye focus for this Mantra: Sit in Easy Pose with a straight spine, pulling in the chin slightly with Neck Lock. Bring the tip of your Jupiter, or index, finger to the tip of your thumb in Giān Mudra, and focus the eyes at the Third Eye Point.[4]

Yogi Bhajan spoke of the Long Ek Ong Kār as follows: "All Mantras are good and are for the awakening of the Divine. But this Mantra is effective and is the Mantra for this time. So my lovely student, at the will of my Master, I teach you the greatest Divine key. It has eight levers and can open the lock of the time, which is also of the vibration of eight. Therefore, when this Mantra is sung with the Neck Lock, at the point where the Prāna and Apāna meet Shushmana, this vibration opens the lock, and thus one becomes one with the Divine."[5]

Kundalini Yoga has a number of Mantras with eight sounds. These create a rhythm that stimulates and nourishes each Chakra.

WĀH YANTĪ — CREATIVITY

wāh yantī, kar yantī, jag dut patī, ādak it wāhā,
brahmāday trayshā gurū, it wāhegurū.

Great Macroself, Creative Self.
All that is creative through time, all that is the Great One.
Three aspects of God: Brahma (Generator), Vishnu (Organizer), Shiva (Deliverer)
That is Wāhegurū.[6]

- wāh yantī: Great Macroself; how cosmic energy and ecstasy is contained within the Inner Self and all-encompassing Cosmic Self

- wāh: ecstasy; the Great Macroself; the larger, unbounded ecstasy

- yantī: from *yantar*; instrument; it is the yantī, which is the mystical diagram that connects our Inner Self with the all-encompassing Cosmic Self of the Universe

- kar yantī: Creative Self (kar: to do, to make; that which does, makes, or creates; yantī: see above)

- jag dut patī: all that is creative through time (jag: world; dut: messenger, envoy, angel of death; patī: husband, Lord, Master)

- ādak it wāhā: all that is the Great One (ād/ādak: etc., so on, and others [adverb]; it: in or with this world; wāhā: manifestation of ecstatic consciousness)

- brahmāday trayshā gurū: three aspects of God—Brahma, Vishnu, Mahesh (Shiva); (brahamaad: Brahma and the other gods; trayshā gurū: the three-part Gurū, the three aspects of God: Generator, Organizer, and Destroyer)

- it wāhegurū: that is Wāhegurū

This second Mantra, Wāh Yantī, opens the way for creativity and cosmic energy. When I sit down to play the music for this Mantra, several different tunes flow through me. Rishi Patanjali offered this Sanskrit Mantra over three thousand years ago; it describes the experience of Wāhegurū. Also called the Gur Mantra, I have always found Wāhegurū an incredible Mantra of transformation, the kind that works so well on the spot when all else has failed. So, in Patanjali's beautiful exploration of Wāhegurū, we essentially get two Mantras in one!

In the first part of this Mantra, Patanjali tells us what "wāhā" means—essentially, "wāh"—ecstasy and expansion, the willingness to go beyond the Inner Self and dive into the reality that is the Cosmic Self of the Universe. Additionally, this acts as the key to connect with the "yantī"—the instrument, or cosmic diagram, that sets in place the relationship of the Inner Self and the Cosmic Self. The relationship between them has always been there, just perhaps not connected from top to bottom, left and right. We come into alignment once again when we chant these words. In alignment, we feel the expansion of the Cosmic Self and experience the capacity to live and remain in Love no matter what. We see everything as the activity and will of the Divine, the One Creator, within and around us all—this is the "kar." Seeing everything this way keeps us in harmony with the Doer, and we accept the Will of the Divine, the flow of the day, and even a simple thing like the direction of a particular conversation. We come to realize how much this God, this beautiful God of ours, loves us so much, and we understand that day after day God sends us lessons to learn and grow, as well as opportunities to burn off our karma and live in our Dharma. Once we realize this, we have experienced "kar yantī"—the way the Divine works and flows within us and the Cosmos.

Then we come to "jag dut patī." We experience a beginning and an end to this life; we are subject to the laws of time and space, time and time again. "Jag" is the world, and "dut" means the messenger of death. However, this Mantra gives us liberation in this cycle of birth and death with the term "patī." With each passing moment, we remain in the hands of the Divine Husband Lord "Patī," and he takes us into His Heart and His Love. This is how the saintly martyrs of the human race face death—with love, devotion, and even exaltation. Think of Jesus on the cross. Think of Gurū Arjan on the hot plate. Think of yourself and the last time you stood up for truth without any hesitation or fear.

So, "wāhā" means this capacity to expand into "wāh" and feel the action of the Divine in "kar," all through the mechanism of the "yantī" that connects our Inner Self with the Cosmic Self, throughout time and space, or "jag dut patī."

Now for the second part of the Mantra. Even after the death of a great saint and martyr and the awakening that comes from tremendous acts of sacrifice, we continue on as mere humans, falling back into the spinning motion of our minds. How could we do anything else? We are made of spinning atoms! So we spin, every day. One thousand thoughts generated in the blink of an eye! And yet even in this chaos we still try, grow, love, search, and find union with the Divine. How do we do it? How do we know that God is real? How do we rise above the anxiety of time and space in the chaos of all this spinning? The answer lies in "brahmāday traysha gurū."

"Brahmāday" is a way of saying "Brahma, Vishnu, and Shiva." Brahma generates, Vishnu experiences or organizes, and Shiva delivers; that is our G.O.D., God. Everything must take birth, everything must experience, and everything must be delivered. Once we understand this, we can experience each lesson with purity, grace, and—ultimately—victory. It doesn't really matter what happens, where you live, who did what, who said what, and on and on. What matters is you. What matters is how you generated truth, organized it, and delivered it. What matters is how you let your attachments go and simply exist in the flow of the Will of the Divine. To experience this capacity requires the Traysha Guru, the Gurū of these three qualities: generation, organization, and delivery. And that is Wāhegurū; that is exactly what Wāhegurū does. Or, as the Mantra says, "it wāhegurū."

As Yogi Bhajan taught: "There are three powers: Brahma, Vishnu, Mahesh. We have their Mantra. Whosoever can recite this Mantra sub-consciously or unconsciously can create these three things at will. Try to understand the power of these words. You know, once the Mantra comes to you, subconsciously or unconsciously, and you become your Mantra, it's called siddh, then you can create all things at will."[7]

THE MŪL MANTRA — INNER TRUTH

ek ong kār, satinām, karatā purakh,
nirbha-u, nirvair, akāl mūrat, ajūnī, saibhang,
gur prasād, jap!
ād sach, jugād sach, hai bhī sach, nānak hosī bhī sach.

God is One, Truth is God's Name, God is the Doer, without fear or vengeance, Undying Form, Unborn, Self-illumined, Gurū's gift, repeat! True in the beginning, true through the ages, true even now, oh Nānak, God is forever true.[8]

- ek: one; the One vibration within all of us

- ong: manifested vibration of the Divine; the creative sound current from which all Creation arises

- kār: to do, to make; that which does, makes, or creates

- satinām: Truth is God's Name, truth I am (sat: the vibration of truth; nām: the Name of God that vibrates through all beings and is what creates us; nām is a noun, that creative vibration that is within; "I am, I am" is the essence of nām)

- karatā purakh: God is the Doer (karatā: the doer; purakh: the Being)

- nirbha-u: without fear

- nirvair: without revenge

- akāl mūrat: Undying Form (akāl: undying; mūrat: image)

- ajūnī: not going through the womb; not subject to birth and death

- saibhang: Self-illumined

- gur prasād: Gurū's gift

- jap: repeat

- ād sach: true in the primal beginning (ād: primal; sach: truth)

- jugād sach: true through the ages (jugād: through the ages; sach: truth)

- hai bhī sach: true even in this moment (hai: he, she, it is; bhī: even)

- nānak hosī bhī sach: Nānak it shall ever be true (nānak: never say no, says Nānak; the energy of Nānak goes into

Universal consciousness where we do not resist reality; hosī:
it shall be; bhī: even; sach: truth)

The Third Mantra, the Mūl Mantra, connects you to the Infinite Truth
beyond questions and boundaries. With boundless energy, this Mantra
corrects misleading thoughts and ideas; without your realizing it, this
Mantra works to align you with truth. You simply vibrate with its eternal truth and relax; doing so, you can discriminate between reality and
falsehood. After his Jal Samādhi, or merger with the One in the water,
Gurū Nānak immediately taught the Mūl Mantra—the first part of Jap
Jī. I think it's a phenomenal blessing that we can practice this Mantra
every day!

I recommend connecting to the Mūl Mantra by taking the meaning of the words and applying them to your life. Allow "ek ong kār" to
bring you into the awareness that God, who is One, exists within all
beings (including you, of course, but also all those who regularly provide you with challenges). Consider the following:

- satinām: Truth is God's Name. The yogīs, saints, and sages
  tell us that all creation emanates from the vibration of
  God's Name. So as God's Name vibrates, we come into
  existence; the sound creates the noun—the "I am," the
  "nām." When we chant "satinām," we are really chanting
  "Truth I am," or "Truth is my identity." We affirm that
  truth prevails. Tap into your inner truth—know it, live by
  it, and be it.

- karatā purakh: God is the Doer. When you understand
  this, life becomes God's dance, God's grace, God's doing.
  Knowing this, you can relax. Yogi Bhajan used to joke that
  in life we simply need a tasty bag of popcorn and a Coke;
  then we can just sit back and enjoy the show.

- nirbha-u: To live without fear. Nirvair: to live without
  anger. There's nothing wrong with fear and anger, we just
  have to acknowledge them and take a deeper look within
  as they arise. Ask your soul what these experiences mean;

investigate what transformation they speak to. As you chant the Mūl Mantra, the words create a purification of fire on the altar of your soul to help you let go of fear and anger and all the other pains that keep you from the pathway of self-healing and love.

- akāl mūrat: Be as God, the undying form. We received this incredible gift of human life and carry within us the infinite nature of the soul. By dressing and living with Grace, we acknowledge the Infinite within us—the undying form manifested in and through us.

- ajūnī: We live beyond the constraints of birth and death and tap into the timeless energy within. We live for legacy and serve the future.

- saibhang: The Self-illumined will of your spirit; the twinkle in your eye and the inner smile that brings you hope in the face of misery. By tapping into God within ourselves, we find the personal freedom to obtain inspiration and dignity at will. We become "saibhang."

- gur prasād: The Gurū's grace, the hand of the Divine that brings us liberation. It guides and cares for us, seeing every moment, witnessing every thought, and lovingly takes us deeper and deeper within ourselves with each life lesson. We acknowledge that we need the help of the Gurū, no matter what form He or She takes: Buddha, Mohammed, Jesus, Mother Mary, Gurū Nānak, and so on.

- jap: Repeat! We repeat the loving Name of God in our chanting, shifting our cellular structure to a Divine resonance.

- ād sach, jugād sach, hai bhī sach, nānak hosī bhī sach: God is true. Divinity is true. Spirituality is true. Switch your understanding and free yourself from the brainwashing of Western culture that reduces spirituality to something only concerning the overtly religious and even then relegates spirituality to something that occurs only on one day of the week. Break the spell; feel and know that Divinity lives in everyone at every time! As Yogi Bhajan says, "That's what you are. You are true in the beginning, true through time, true now, and you shall be true, if you remain so, but you don't remain so. You want to be something else. Be what God made you to be."[9]

SAT SIRĪ SIRĪ AKĀL — BEYOND DEATH

sat sirī, sirī akāl, sirī akāl, mahā akāl,
mahā akāl, satinām, akāl mūrat, wāhegurū.

True and Great One, Great Undying One, Great Undying One, Exalted One, Undying One, Exalted One, Undying One, Truth is God's Name, Undying Form, great is the experience of Gurū; that One who brings us from darkness (gu) to light (rū).[10]

- sat sirī: True and Great One (sat: truth; sirī: great)

- sirī akāl (said twice): Great Spirit, Undying One (sirī: great; akāl: undying)

- mahā akāl (said twice): Exalted One, Undying One (mahā: exalted One; akāl: undying)

- satinām: Truth is God's Name (sat: the vibration of truth; nām: the Name of God that creates and vibrates through us all; "I am, I am"—the essence of nām)

- akāl mūrat: undying form (akāl: undying; mūrat: image)

- wāhegurū: ecstatic (Wāh!) is the experience of the Gurū, that which takes us from darkness to light.

The fourth Mantra, Sat Sirī Sirī Akāl, serves as the Mantra for the Aquarian Age. It gives us the capacity to relate to the Infinite nature of the Soul. Here I capitalize *Soul* to emphasize that the inner vibration of the Soul works in complete concert, connection, and identity with the Great Cosmic Soul, the Divine within all beings, or as some say, God. This connection means we are deathless, timeless. This Mantra affirms the possibility of living our lives with an awareness of this Infinity. Our actions become not only about our own lives, but about everyone's lives. When we tap into the Soul and its infinite nature, we can live without fear. We can see the truth, know the truth, and live the truth. In this way we leave a legacy so that the generations to follow will be served by our presence here on Earth. The penetration of this Mantra guides our lives on a day-to-day basis so that we take the right course and abide in the Infinite Flow, allowing us to merge with the One at the time of death. When we vibrate with the Infinite, we become the Infinite; when we vibrate with the finite, we become the finite. When we chant this Mantra, we affirm the energy and connection to the Undying One—the undying nature of the Divine, the undying nature of the Soul. We worship and merge with it.

We begin with "sat sirī, sirī akāl, sirī akāl, mahā akāl, mahā akāl!"—True and Great One, great Undying One, Great Undying One, Exalted One, Undying One, Exalted One, Undying One! And then we chant "satinām," meaning Truth is God's Name. As with the Mūl Mantra, this also means, "Truth I am." So in the course of this Mantra, we praise the Infinite nature of the One, and then we affirm that Infinite nature within ourselves. Then we end with "akāl mūrat, wāhegurū." This acknowledges the Undying Form again, and calls upon the Gurū to take us into union.

In this way we give ourselves the tool, the method, the way to experience each moment in our highest consciousness and wisdom. The Undying Form for us is within the Shabad Gurū, the vibration of chanting God's Name. In this way, we find our way to move forward, our way to heal every moment, our way to find the light in every situation, and our way to live. Wāhegurū!

Yogi Bhajan said, "Satinām is your back, your Earth, your spine. Wāhegurū is your face, God is your front."[11] This Mantra perfectly gives us the experience of this incredible and powerful method, or breast stroke, of "satinām" as our back and "wāhegurū" as our front. If you look at the Mantra, we first connect with "satinām" as our identity, and then with "wāhegurū" as our method to attain union with the

Divine. I use this metaphor of a swimmer because that is what we are doing—swimming through life!

In our day-to-day lives, it is easy and natural to relate to and therefore be attached to the play of the world: work, school, family, children. All of these things are important no doubt, yet when we lose our connection to that which feeds the Soul, there is a whole level of reality and self-fulfillment that is at a sum total loss in our being. What is it that we lose when we do not relate to the undying nature of the Soul? I want to relate a story from H. H. Pujya Swami Chidanand Saraswatiji about a student of a spiritual teacher; it's helped me answer the question for myself.[12]

There once lived a devoted student who meditated with a lot of dedication. One day the student met with his spiritual teacher and said, "You know, sir, I love this spiritual path, but I also want to get married and have a family life. May I have your permission to do so?"

The master said, "Sure, go ahead; I will come for you in ten years."

The student got married to a lovely lady and had three children. After ten years the spiritual teacher came and knocked on the student's door. The student answered and immediately dropped to his knees. "Please," he begged, "let me stay another ten years. My children are young and my wife needs my support."

"Okay," said the sage.

Another ten years passed and the spiritual teacher returned. Yet again the student pleaded, "Sir, my children are going to college. I must make enough money to support them. Please can I have another ten years?"

So ten more years passed. The spiritual teacher returned to his student's house, which looked quite opulent with a lot of additions. Outside, a fierce-looking dog stood guard. But the spiritual teacher recognized the dog as the Soul of his student. The man had suffered an accidental death, and—due to his longing to protect his home—came back as a guard dog. The dog immediately recognized his master and licked his hand. But in that moment, too, he asked his teacher for ten more years. "Soon my children will have children of their own. Who will protect them and all of the wealth we have built up?"

The spiritual teacher gave his consent and left. Ten more years passed, and this time the spiritual teacher could tell with his intuition that his student had become a cobra intent on guarding the family safe, hidden in one of the walls of the house. Various children ran around the yard and the sage called to them.

"Please go and get me the cobra that lives in the wall. You'll find him wrapped around the safe. Break his back. Don't worry, he will not hurt you."

And so the children did as the master requested—they found the cobra, broke his back, and brought him to the spiritual teacher. The sage held the cobra by his neck and began the long walk back to his ashram. He said, "I'm sorry that I had to break your back, but the time has come for you to connect with the Infinity of your spirit. You were lost in increasing attachment to this Earth, and I had to break the cycle."

"Sat Sirī Sirī Akāl" speaks to our need to live as householders—to get married, to keep jobs, and to raise children in such a way that we connect with the Infinite nature of the Soul every day. We have a unique opportunity with this Mantra to manifest and master the concept of "Jiwan Mukht"—liberated while alive. This connection to our Infinite nature helps us become better mothers, better fathers, more intimate lovers, more present with our families, more effective and authentic in our work, and more energized for life; in the end, it also helps us let all of this go. "Let go and let God," as Yogi Bhajan would say.[13] With this Mantra, we affirm that every moment matters. That every moment serves as an opportunity to live in the consciousness of the undying One.

RAKHAY RAKHANAHĀR — PROTECTION

rakhay rakhanahār āp ubāri-an, gur kī pairī pā-i kāj savāri-an,
ho-ā āp da-i-āl manah(u) na visāri-an, sādh janā kai
sang bhavajal tāri-an,
sākat nindak dusht khin mā-he bidāri-an,
tis sāhib kī tayk nānak manai mā-he,
jis simarat sukh ho-i sagalay dūkh jā-he.

The Great Protector, the One who protects, that One who exists within us of Himself or Herself lifts us up. That One gave us the Lotus Feet of the Gurū on our foreheads and so all of our affairs and work

*are taken care of. God is merciful, kind, and compassionate so that we
do not forget God in our mind. In the company of the Holy, we are
carried across the challenges, calamities, and scandals of the world.
Attachment to the world and slanderous enemies are destroyed. That
great Lord is my anchor. Nānak, keep firm in your mind and cultivate
the vibration of peace by meditating and repeating God's Name, and
all happiness comes while sorrows and pain go away.*[14]

- rakhay rakhaṇahār āp ubāri-an: the Great Protector,
  the One who protects, that One who exists within us of
  Himself or Herself lifts us up (rakh: to protect, look after;
  rakhaṇahār: the agent who protects; āp: Himself, Itself,
  Yourself, Myself, of the Self; ubāri-an: to deliver across)

- gur kī pairī pā-i kāj savāri-an: that One gave us the Lotus
  Feet of the Gurū on our foreheads and so all of our affairs
  and work are taken care of (gur: the Gurūship, source of
  wisdom, and source of inspiration; kī: of; pairī: foot; pā-i:
  obtain; kāj: work, task, wedding; savāri-an: set in order,
  arrange, set right, adjust, adorn)

- ho-ā āp da-i-āl manah(u) na visāri-an: God is merciful,
  kind, and compassionate as we do not forget God in our
  minds (ho-ā: is; āp: Himself, Itself, Yourself, Myself, of the
  Self; da-i-āl: kindness, mercy, compassion; manah(u): from
  the mind; na: not; visāri-an: forget)

- sādh janā kai sang bhavajal tāri-an: in the company of the
  Holy we are carried across the challenges, calamities, and
  scandals of the world (sādh janā: saintly people; kai sang: with;
  bhavajal: world ocean; tāri-an: to swim across, maneuver)

- sākat nindak dusht khin mā-he bidāri-an: attachment to the
  world, slander, and evil are destroyed in an instant (sākat:
  devotion to the world, worldly person; nindak: slandering;
  dusht: as adjective it means "wicked, evil, bad"; as noun it
  means "evil person, enemy, wretch"; khin: instant; mā-he:
  in; bidāri-an: tear to pieces, destroy)

• tis sāhib kī ṭayk nānak manai mā-he: that great Lord is my
anchor in Nānak's mind (tis sāhib: such a Lord; kī ṭayk: the
master's support, reliance, trust; nānak manai: in Nānak's
mind; mā-he: in)

• jis simarat sukh ho-i sagalay dūkh jā-he: in remembering
all happiness comes while sorrows and pain go away
(jis: who; simarat: remembrance, meditation; sukh ho-i:
peace comes into being; sagalay: all; dūkh: troubles; jā-he:
depart) Nānak's mind is full of the support and trust
of God, whose vibration is peace, so all troubles simply
depart—there's no room for trouble anymore!

The Fifth Gurū, Gurū Arjan, gave us this fifth Mantra, Rakhay
Rakhaṇahār. It provides protection for us and our entire community. When accompanying this sweet Mantra, musicians often choose
beautiful, lyrical tunes because of the energy that this Mantra evokes.
However, the effect of the Mantra is more like a sword wielded by the
fiercest warrior you could imagine. This combination of both sweet
and fierce protects our innocence.

Gurū Arjan compiled the writings of the Sikh Gurūs and other saints
to make the Ādī Granth, and completed the construction of the Golden
Temple, one of the most sacred Gurdwārās for Sikhs today. He accom-
plished these monumental tasks with tremendous humility and love, all
while enduring negativity from his jealous brother and, eventually, the
Emperor of India. As I relayed before, the Emperor tortured Gurū Arjan,
but he remained serene and meditative through the whole experience.
This incredible example reminds us to stand strong, remain peaceful, and
keep in union with the One no matter what. Sometimes we get caught
up in a victim mindset and try to assign blame for all the challenging
things happening to us, as opposed to just identifying the energy for what
it is. When we act this way, the negative energy tends to build as we fuel
it with our own distress. Through his equipoise and inner peace, Gurū
Arjan neutralized the negative energy because he remained within the
fortress of Inner Truth—he received everything without reacting. All
present—including the Emperor—realized they were witnessing the
actions of a saint.

After so much torture, and according to the will of the Divine, Gurū Arjan left his body. A few years later, his son, Gurū Hargobind, took up the sword and secured freedom for the Sikhs and others in the region. Although the Rakhay Rakhaṇahār Mantra of protection comes from Gurū Arjan, Gurū Hargobind delivered security and protection on the physical plane. In the same way, we may not experience the effects of a Mantra in this lifetime; it may take generations for the benefit to manifest. So just chant, chant, chant, with no desires, and no need for immediate outcome. What resonates within us is Spirit, which lies beyond time and space. In the end, it is Spirit, and Spirit alone, that is nurtured by these Mantras.

WĀHEGURŪ WĀHE JĪ-O — VICTORY

wāhegurū, wāhegurū, wāhegurū, wāhe jī-o.

Ecstatic (Wāh!) is the experience of the Gurū, that One who brings us from darkness (gu) to light (rū). Ecstatic (Wāh!) is the experience of the Jī-o, the soul within that connects with the Divine Cosmic Soul of the One.[15]

- wāhegurū: ecstatic (Wāh!) is the experience of the Gurū, that which takes us from darkness to light

- wāhe jī-o: ecstatic is the experience of the Jī-o: the soul within connecting to the Divine Cosmic Soul of the One

At this stage of the practice, we go extremely deep into the psyche. We recite this chant for twenty-two minutes—the longest duration for any chant in the Aquarian Sādhanā—so there's plenty of time to get into it, enjoy it, and then become thoroughly bored with it. And that's when it takes hold of us. In this moment of boredom, if we stay with it and allow the rhythm of the words to keep pulsing throughout our consciousness, the Gurū will come in and lift us to a place where the mind no longer holds any domain—we enter a space that is between us, our soul, and the vibratory frequency of our own consciousness.

Think of this practice as the journey of a smooth black stone thrown into the water. The eye focus at the tip of the nose shows the pathway for the stone to sink deeper. Each repetition of "wāhegurū" clears the subconscious of the negativity from within and around us. The stone creates ripples and waves rise up; the boat gets rocked! Transformation occurs. Everything about you will feel it—your home, your family, your life. Keep chanting "wāhegurū." Although the ripples and waves may seem rough at first, in time you go deeper and deeper into the waters of the self.

Then we chant "wāhe-jī-o": the sweetness of the Mantra. It brings us the gift of the Jī, the soul, which means to search and fall in love with the Beloved, God Himself, Herself, Itself. This kind of falling in love has no end and no limit. As the stone sinks to the very depths of your being, you remain in deep meditation.

To aid in our journey inward, we have the assistance of a very powerful posture called *Virāsan*. This is the only chant in the Aquarian Sādhanā that employs this posture. It can be intimidating at first, but let me just explain a bit about the posture, ways to support yourself with props, and the amazing benefits you can obtain from it.

Virāsan

Keep your hands in Prayer Pose, bringing your left palm and right palm together at the heart center. Sit on your left heel with it placed on your perineum and the right knee close to the chest. This should straighten your spine. Instead of collapsing your left foot, you can use padding to comfortably maintain the correct position. I like to use two pillows: one between the top of my foot and the floor, and the other between my heel and perineum. If you sit with the flat part of your foot turned out and the spine crooked, you will end up tipping to one side.[16] By sitting on the left heel like this, we open the connection between the first and seventh Chakras so that the Kundalini can rise. With the right knee up, we put pressure on the liver for purification and courage.[17] As well, we have the capacity to stand up quickly from this posture for action, symbolizing that we live as warrior saints in this world. With our hands in

Virāsan

Prayer Pose, we embody a state of humility, and with our eyes focused at the tip of the nose, we go beyond the ego and the mind.

Vir means hero. *Āsan* means posture. So this is a hero's posture. This posture was especially practiced during the time of Gurū Gobind Singh, the tenth Gurū of the Sikhs, when Emperor Aurangzeb of India forcibly tried to convert people to his religion. Although it meant death to stand up to the Emperor, that's exactly what Gurū Gobind Singh did. During the spring festival of Baisākhī in 1699, he called Sikhs from all over India to gather in Anandpur Sāhib. Thousands attended the gathering. Gurū Gobind Singh raised his sword and addressed them.

"Who will give me your head?" he asked.

A wave of shock went through the crowd and all remained silent, until one Sikh stood up and proclaimed, "My head has always been yours."

Gurū Gobind Singh took the man to the tent behind the stage. The crowd heard the sound of a sword cutting through flesh, and Gurū Gobind Singh emerged with his bloody weapon. Once again, he asked the same question of the assembled crowd. Some people fled, others watched in dismay. Another Sikh offered his head to Gurū Gobind Singh, and once again he took the man behind the stage and came back with fresh gore on his weapon. This scenario was repeated three more times. However, after the last time, instead of emerging from the tent with a bloody sword, Gurū Gobind Singh came out with the five Sikhs who had given him their heads.

The five men wore new clothes, dressed as rajas of the time. Gurū Gobind Singh dressed them this way, calling this royal clothing *Bānā*. In addition to the beautiful clothing, the men's faces radiated; they beamed with blessings from the Gurū and their internal process of surrender. Gurū Gobind Singh and the five Sikhs began to prepare *Amrit* (divine nectar), which is prepared by chanting as one stirs a Kirpān (steel sword) in water that is held in a steel bowl. Mātā Sāhib Kaur (Gurū Gobind Singh's wife) poured sugar into the water to infuse the liquid with the qualities of kindness and love. With the entrancing sound of steel on steel, the assembled sang sacred recitations *(Bāṇīs)*. All five men sat in Virāsan during this time for at least an hour. Once fully prepared, the Guru gave the Amrit to them. Each pledged to live with purity of heart and soul as taught by Gurū Gobind Singh.

He gave all women the name Kaur, which means princess. To men, Gurū Gobind Singh gave the name Singh, which means lion. By doing so, he conveyed that royalty, divinity, and grace do not come with one's standing at birth; they arise from our own sense of self-worth, honor, and integrity. In this way, Gurū Gobind Singh taught us to crown ourselves as kings and queens, and by doing so, he stood up to the Emperor in a timeless way. No matter our religion or lifestyle, let us all live in the royalty of the heart!

Then, in an act of profound humility, Gurū Gobind Singh assumed the Virāsan pose and asked the five Sikhs to offer him the Amrit. He completely surrendered himself; the Gurū and the disciple became one. Before this time, he was named Gurū Gobind Rai; after he was known as Gurū Gobind Singh. Twenty thousand Sikhs took Amrit on that day. The community eventually rose up in battle against the Mogul Empire, becoming an essential part of the end of its radical reign.

ਵਾਹ ਵਾਹ ਗੋਬਿੰਦ ਸਿੰਘ ਆਪੇ ਗੁਰੁ ਚੇਲਾ ॥੧॥

wāh wāh gobind singh āpay gur chaylā. || 1||

Hail Hail Gurū Gobind Singh, the Gurū and the Disciple are one!

BHAI GURDĀS JĪ, *AMRIT KĪRTAN*[18]

As Yogi Bhajan explained, "Gurū and disciple became one. Finite and infinity became one. Karma and Dharma became one. Life and death became one. And Gurū gave us Wāheguru as our Gurū."[19]

The posture of Virāsan and the Mantra Wāheguru Wāhe Jī-o enable us to surrender to the Will of the Divine and emerge victorious. We might not have actual swords, but we each can live like warriors by living in integrity with our words and actions, standing up for truth in whatever way we can.

GURŪ RĀM DĀS CHANT — GRACE AND HUMILITY

gurū gurū wāheguru, gurū rām dās gurū.

This is in praise of the consciousness of Gurū Rām Dās, invoking his spiritual light, guidance, and protective grace. We are filled with humility.[20]

- gurū gurū wāhegurū: as we chant this, we call out to the Cosmos, reaching up through the ladder, or the doorway of Gurū (gurū: that One who brings us from darkness [gu] to light [rū]; wāhegurū: ecstatic [Wāh!] is the experience of the Gurū, that which takes us from darkness to light)

- gurū rām dās gurū: Gurū Rām Dās, the servant of God, comes to serve us (gurū: that One who brings us from darkness [gu] to light [rū]; rām: God; dās: servant of God)

Finally, we chant the seventh Mantra to Gurū Rām Dās at the end of Sādhanā to receive his healing energy. You do not have to be a Sikh or a religious person at all to relate to Gurū Rām Dās: he simply represents the energy of compassion, love, and healing in the Universe. You can tune in to these qualities and know that somewhere, someplace, all Masters, Saints, Sages, and Gurūs come from the same source. It depends on where you live, of course, but we usually arrive at this chant at first light—the sun might even be rising, which is the most appropriate time for this Mantra. It includes our innermost prayers, the ones we don't even know exist—the prayers that come from our soul.

When we chant "gurū gurū wāhegurū," we reach out to the Cosmos, in essence asking for transformation. If you wish to avoid transformation, you should avoid this chant! Remember that the word "Gurū" means he or she who guides us from darkness (gu) to light (rū); the Gurū brings us completely into our own consciousness. By chanting "gurū gurū," we reach out to that particular agent or energy of change. The Gurū acts as the Hand of God, lifting us up. When we chant "wāhegurū," we accept the transformation. "Come what may, whatever change you have in store for me, oh Lord, I welcome it in the highest bliss and ecstasy of my soul, Wāh!" And so we embrace the change and enjoy it. We eat it for breakfast!

When we chant "gurū rām dās gurū," the energy of the Cosmos comes to serve us with the words "rām dās," which means servant (dās) of God (rām). We create a direct communication with the Divine, asking for answers, clarity, and a sense of direction. This communication alone stirs the Divine to respond to the vibration of the call, which we may experience in overt ways—for example, we attain sudden clarity about a particular personal issue or maybe we simply feel better. Sometimes in just feeling better, we can rise above the challenges of the day, see them more clearly, and engage with them without our habitual entanglement. Instead, we allow our daily trials to change us, bringing us to a purer sense of Self and Love within.

As you might guess, Gurū Rām Dās—the fourth Gurū of the Sikhs (also called the Lord of Miracles)—is the guardian of this Mantra. Personally, this Mantra often acts as a kind of spiritual forklift—it raises me up out of any dark place and places me into the natural radiant stillness at the center of my being. It truly works! Sometimes I chant this Mantra for five minutes, and everything totally shifts; sometimes it takes a couple of hours. I simply chant and wait for the Mantra to do its work, releasing my worries, ego, and fear into the Cosmic flow of the Gurū.

I remember a particular concert in Seattle: We had just finished, and the hall remained packed with people. The incredible energy of chanting still permeated through all of us, and the lights inside emitted an almost surreal golden hue, a color chosen by the angels to accompany this moment of joy that we were all experiencing. Through the laughter and chatter, I hopped down from the stage and prepared to make my way through the crowd. Suddenly, a man in his eighties stopped me. His dark brown eyes pierced through the light.

"Do you have a Mantra for depression?" he asked.

Thinking that I misheard him, I asked him to repeat himself.

"Do you have a Mantra for depression?" He was serious. From the intense look in his dark brown eyes, I could tell he was referring to his own depression.

I had no idea what to say. What could I tell this elder? How could I respond to honor the pain within him, to actually help? I closed my eyes and prayed to Gurū Rām Dās. What should I say? I implored. What's the answer?

And then the answer came: Gurū gurū wāhegurū, gurū rām dās guru. Tell him. Tell him this Mantra will relieve depression.

So I opened my eyes and looked into his and told him to chant this Mantra. It was one of those wonderful moments in my life, where as I said the words I knew they were utterly true.

A MOMENT OF SILENCE

Please take a few minutes at the end of the Aquarian Mantras to sit in silence, allowing the resonance of the chants to soak in, allowing the energy of the practice to vibrate within, and silently connecting with the Divine. I find that this time of morning is perfect for connecting in silence. In silence we find answers, feel complete, and know the song of the Universe before it unfolds in the new day.

Silence

Nothing to do.

Nothing to be.

Empty.

Nothing to ask for.

Nothing to need.

Silence.

That is God.

That is me.

That is Thee.

Chapter Eight

SURRENDER, BOW, AND RECEIVE

Stage Five: Gateway to Divinity

ਨਾਨਕੁ ਨਾਮ ਚੜਦੀ ਕਲਾ

nānak nām charadī kalā

Through Nānak may Thy Name forever increase and the spirit be exalted,

ਤੇਰੇ ਭਾਣੇ ਸਰਬੱਤ ਦਾ ਭਲਾ ॥

tayray bhāṇay sarabat dā bhalā.

And may all people prosper by Thy Grace.

FROM THE *ARDĀS (DAILY PRAYER) OF THE SIKH TRADITION*[1]

As a teenager I had a crush on this guy. He didn't share the same feelings but let me know in a nice way. Yet, ouch! It hurt. To process the pain, I wrote a poem and tucked it away in some dark drawer. The poem went something like this:

> I have fallen at your door
>
> And yet it does not open

After my morning practice the next day, I did an Ardās (the Sikh traditional standing prayer), followed by a Hukam. I can't recall the exact phrasing of the reading, but it went something like this:

"Oh child of God, you have come to the sanctuary of the Gurū's door, and that door is always open."

Alone in the Gurdwārā, which served as our family meditation room, I dropped my head and wept. The tears fell and fell. My shoulders shook, and I wailed. And then I laughed. Oh, how loved I truly was! I had found the right door to fall down in front of.

In the final stage of Sādhanā, we pray and give our practice back to the Divine by bowing our head to something greater than us. We come to the door of that One who can lift us up, and then we bow and enter into the heart of this space. Once inside, we have the capacity to listen to what the Divine has to say to us. Bringing the practice back to the Divine balances our energy and keeps us in a place of service and humility throughout the day.

In the Sikh tradition we practice the final stage of the Aquarian Sādhanā in a Gurdwārā, our sanctuary. You'll find more information in this chapter about Gurdwārā if you are so inclined to participate or just want to gain more knowledge about our practices. In addition, I also talk about a method of connecting to the Gurū if you do not have the capacity to set up a Gurdwārā space.

If you prefer to stay within your tradition, here are three universal acts of consciousness that I invite you to apply that are key in this stage of the Aquarian Sadhānā:

1. **Bow.** By bowing, we bring our head lower than the heart, thus setting the frequency of the day—we hold the heart (our courage, joy, and freedom) above the head (our thoughts and various mental struggles), and we offer this to the Divine. After all of our practice and the raising of the Kundalini, we give all that energy back to the Divine in a state of humility by bowing. To truly understand, we must "stand under," as I remember Yogi Bhajan saying. In this act of bowing, we humble ourselves and ask the Divine Will what it wants of us. We "stand under" life itself and ask how we can serve. We may not always like the answer that we receive, but if we truly bow, we will experience no resistance to that Divine inner river that flows through us. Bowing is an opportunity

to say yes to that flow and truly let our dramas and traumas go because we see their smallness in comparison to this penetrating light of Divine energy simply waiting for us to bow and receive it into our lives.

2. **Pray.** Our prayers give the opportunity for our soul's longing to be heard, for our highest intentions to come forward, and for a conversation with the Divine to open up in our lives.

3. **Take a Divine reading.** You can ask the Divine to speak to you with a sacred reading. Everything in the previous four stages of the Aquarian Sādhanā prepared you to hear the Divine voice. I invite you to welcome this voice through the Bhagavad Gita, the Torah, the Koran, the Bible, your favorite book of poems, or any other text you hold as sacred. Feel the vibration of the Holy as you take this reading. Know that the Divine speaks to you through this reading and let the words guide you for the rest of the day. Do this on a regular basis and the real magic will start to kick in.

THE GURDWĀRĀ EXPERIENCE

Gurdwārā means gateway or door (dwārā) to the Guru. Gurdwārā is a sacred space centered around the Siri Guru Granth Sāhib, a sacred text compiled by the fifth Guru of the Sikhs, Guru Arjan. This sacred space is held within either a single room for a family Gurdwārā or in a temple space for larger community gatherings. When entering a Gurdwārā, we cover our head and take our shoes off, and in some Gurdwārās, we have the opportunity to wash our hands and feet.

Before the tenth Guru of the Sikhs, Guru Gobind Singh, left his body, he empowered the Siri Guru Granth Sāhib to serve as the living Guru. I don't even think of it as a "text" because it holds such a living and breathing place in my life. As discussed before, the writings contained in the Siri Guru Granth Sāhib come from the Sikh Gurus but also from masters of other traditions, in this way honoring the truth that all paths that lead to the Divine are true and real. As Sikhs, we gather in the presence of the Sirī Gurū Granth Sāhib and in doing so feel a quiet, sweet peace that resonates in the air. When we enter the space of the Gurdwārā, we bow our heads to the Sirī Gurū Granth Sāhib, giving all of our problems to the Divine, handing over our egos and offering ourselves in service.

ਦੁਖ ਪਰਹਰਿ ਸੁਖੁ ਘਰਿ ਲੈ ਜਾਇ ॥

dukh parahar sukh ghar lai jā-i.

Having given up sorrow to God, take peace and go home with it.

GURŪ NĀNAK, *FIFTH PAURĪ OF JAP JĪ*[2]

SHABADS

In the presence of the Gurū, we sing Shabads (sacred poems) and celebrate the power of the Shabad Gurū. After everything we've practiced in the Aquarian Sādhanā up to this point, we can now truly experience the Divine energy in a palpable way. The bliss of this is like nectar to the soul. We are not asking for anything; we are just enjoying. Yet the energy becomes enthroned in our hearts, which opens the door to live in harmony with the Divine this day and always. I grew up this way; this is how the energy of the Shabad Gurū found its way into my heart. As we sing these songs together, we celebrate the knowledge that Divinity is real and true. The last track on the *Light of the Naam with Long Ek Ong Kar* CD provided with this book has a Shabad that has brought me great joy and transformation called "Dhan Dhan Rām Dās Gur."

In a full Gurdwārā service, we sing the "Song of the Khālsā." Khālsā means purity—remaining true to the soul and the essential self. As a way to illustrate the basic principles of Khālsā, this song narrates the history of the Sikhs, but you don't have to be a Sikh to benefit from it. Then we recite the first five Paurīs of a sacred poem called "Anand Sāhib," which means Song of Bliss. Reciting these stanzas guides us to bliss by steering us toward relationship with the Divine.

ARDĀS

After these sacred songs, we bow and rise for the Ardās, or prayer. When we state our intentions and goals directly, they become manifested on the planet. And standing is important here: As I remember Yogi Bhajan exclaiming, "We stand up for our prayers!" We stand by our prayers and declare our highest intentions and goals in service to the Divine in all beings.

During the Ardās, we call upon the energy of all ten Sikh Gurūs to come to our aid, to help us feel connected to all those who have lived and died for our Dharma. We ask for unity. We ask to remain in the Divine flow, and we offer our day at the feet of the Divine. We pray for peace on the earth, we pray for healing for those who are ill, and we pray for our community. Often, people write down names in a special notebook for those in need of healing or assistance; we mention these people later in the Ardās, thereby sending them tremendous blessings. After the Ardās, we bow once again.

Bowing repeatedly during the final stage of the Aquarian Sādhanā practice balances the energy of the practice. After the Kundalini has risen through the top of the head, bowing stabilizes our energy for the rest of the day.

HUKAM

Then we take a sacred, spontaneous reading from the Sirī Gurū Granth Sāhib. Actually, "sacred reading" isn't the best translation; a better one is "command." In a meditative way, the person reading from the Gurū surrenders to the Divine and opens to whatever page is meant to be opened. Then the Hukam begins and the subsequent reading pertains to everyone sitting there. I take a Hukam every day, and without fail I receive guidance for living my life in joy, love, and peace. When people express the wish to find a Gurū, someone they can go to for assistance and advice, I realize how lucky I am to have the Sirī Gurū Granth Sāhib, this amazing wealth of wisdom. The advice always comes. You just have to listen.

GUR PRASĀD AND LANGAR

This is the most important part, at least my tummy thinks so! If you have kids or a family and want to create community and enjoy life, take note. At the end of Gurdwārā, we serve a treat infused with prayers called Gur Prasād, made of flour, sugar, clarified butter, and water. As a little girl I always loved finding ways to get as much Gur Prasād as my little tummy could hold. After this sweet delight, we enjoy each other's company, talking and laughing, while the kids run around and wreak havoc. Pure bliss!

A sacred and free meal called Langar is often served. Langar offers a wonderful opportunity for Seva (selfless service) in that we prepare and serve food for whoever joins us.

EXPERIENCING THE ENERGY OF THE GURŪ WITHOUT A GURDWĀRĀ

If you can't do a Gurdwārā with the Sirī Gurū Granth Sāhib properly set up and you would like to connect with the Gurū, try this version:

Make some kind of altar to focus your attention on, or use anything that lifts your spirit—the rising sun, the ocean, mountains, a river, a tree, a flower, or something else! You just need something that helps transport you beyond ego and personality, something that helps you tap into the Divine.

Stand up to do your Ardās. You can use the version I offer in appendix D. After you finish, really bow. Sink into that bow and invite others to do so as well.

After Ardās, take a Hukam right then and there! Try this by opening Jap Jī and reading wherever your eye falls. You can also use an app to download the daily Hukam from the Golden Temple in Amritsar, India.

CLOSING SONG FOR PEOPLE OF ALL FAITHS

To finish the fifth stage of the Aquarian Sādhanā, we sing the song called "Long Time Sun," originally sung by Mike Heron of the Incredible String Band back in the sixties. When Yogi Bhajan first came to teach Kundalini Yoga, he couldn't believe how much neurosis there was in the West. But when he heard "Long Time Sun," he absolutely loved it—if Westerners could come up with such a beautiful song, there must be hope for us yet! So he asked us to chant it after every Kundalini Yoga class and after every Aquarian Sādhanā practice. We sing "Long Time Sun" three times. When we share this song in public, I like to tell people that the first time is for them, the second is for all the people they love, and the third time is for all the people that they don't love! You can find a recorded version of this song on my CD entitled *The Essential Snatam Kaur.*

> May the long time sun shine upon you
>
> All love surround you
>
> And the pure light within you
>
> Guide your way on[3]

Chant *Sat Nām* three times at the end. And, well . . . frankly, with all of this done, you are set for a blessed day ahead for sure.

BRINGING THE DIVINE TO THE EARTH

I once visited a cathedral in Cologne, Germany. It took hundreds of years to build, spanning generations of bishops, architects, builders, and worshippers. Standing there, I realized how incredibly addicted we are to fast results, especially in the West. Even so, we have the capacity to take diligent steps.

Take your time with this final stage; take diligent steps. Set positive intentions and goals, and open your inner ear to the Divine voice. Hearing what the Divine has to say takes a lot of time and effort, maybe even a lifetime of work. However, we're not just limited to our own lifetime—we can actually tap into the lifetimes of dedicated practitioners before us, aligning ourselves with the wisdom of the ages. In this way, we become timeless in our effort to give ourselves back to the Divine. And so, as we start our day, maybe leaving our front door with briefcase in hand, we aren't alone—an army of angels has heard our prayers. Without a doubt, they help us open whatever doors the day brings, along with the hearts of every person we meet. And why shouldn't they? We live in service of the Divine. And if we don't, well . . . this practice will find a way to make sure we do.

~ *Chapter Nine* ~

PRESENCE OF SELF

ਜਿਨੀ ਤੂੰ ਸੇਵਿਆ ਭਾਉ ਕਰਿ ਸੇ ਤੁਧੁ ਪਾਰਿ ਉਤਾਰਿਆ ॥

jin tū sayvi-ā bhā-u kar say tudh pār utāri-ā.

Those who serve You with love are carried across.

SATTA AND BALWAND, *SIRĪ GURŪ GRANTH SĀHIB JĪ*[1]

If you're like me, you can sometimes get overwhelmed by the various demands of life. These are the times to lean on your spiritual practice. Personally, I rely on the Sādhanā to help me find my center and guide me through the challenges; as a result, my practice deepens with each journey. In this chapter I would like to share with you some of my passages through hardships—I hope it assists you through your own.

I also want to ask you to think a bit about yourself and what you need in your life right now to return to your quiet center. From this place of quiet, we can access the presence of self and meet the challenges of the day. We may feel afraid sometimes, but facing hardships directly transforms our experience into one permeated with love and beauty in unexpected ways. Major changes can happen in mere seconds, or they may take decades through daily diligent effort; either way, we can blossom forth into the original light of who we truly are and experience our own mastery.

IDENTIFYING YOUR BOTTOM LINE

For a while, my husband and I lived out of an RV while on tour with our newborn daughter. I felt completely overwhelmed, exhausted, and confused about pretty much everything in my life. I also felt the incredible loving support coming from our new family configuration, but I was still spread pretty thin. I woke up every three hours at night to nurse my daughter, often after staying up until midnight performing. My husband drove us from city to city, caring for our daughter in countless parking lots of seemingly endless concert halls. Before the birth of my daughter, I practiced nearly three hours almost every morning. During this time, however, all of my practice—along with any sense of control—seemed to fly out of the RV's open window as we trekked down yet another highway.

One afternoon as we approached the outskirts of some desert town, I spoke with my life coach on the phone as my daughter napped. I paused after listing off all of my problems.

"You've got to figure out your bottom line," she replied. "What do you absolutely need to maintain your grace and feel centered?"

I closed my eyes, and surprisingly the answer popped right into my head with crystal clarity: I need thirty minutes of yoga every day, no matter what, or I'll go nuts.

"Good!" she responded. "Now you've got to do it."

So the next morning I just did it. While my daughter slept, I just did yoga in our RV bed because there was no other space available and no other time. And you know, it worked! In that craziness of touring, I got my baseline practice in, and that made all the difference. And, of course, things eventually changed, as they always do: my daughter started sleeping through the night, and I returned to my regularly scheduled practice.

Maybe you can't envision having the time or space for spiritual practice. Try to find your bottom line. Maybe everything else has failed—trying to solve your problems by worldly means has only brought you down to rock bottom. That's good news. When we hit rock bottom, we're actually ready for a fantastic paradigm shift. Regardless of where you find yourself, you still need to articulate your bottom line so you can finally climb your way up, one rung at a time. So ask yourself this question: What do I need in my life, every day, to find balance and remain centered?

Everyone will answer this differently. You might be able to identify your bottom line right now in this moment. It might take a life-changing journey for you to discover it. Whatever your bottom line looks like, meeting it is crucial to getting through overwhelming times, staying afloat, and emerging from difficulties into genuine metamorphosis. It's the sweetest victory I have ever known.

PARADIGM SHIFTS

I feel more clear about the purpose of this book than I do about most things in my life. Throughout the years of my incredible musical journey, I have regularly witnessed how people have been touched by the Mantras, yoga, and meditations I've shared. This has kept me going through all of the demands on my time to travel and perform, and I've always known that it isn't just about me. Sometimes the intensity of my schedule literally makes me sick. Sometimes I have to cancel performances, and it breaks my heart. Sometimes my voice gives out, and I can't sing and the audience ends up singing to me! In these moments when I experience the limitations of my physical body, I understand that the Divine will take care of it, just as the Divine has all along. It's not me that comes through for people in an audience; it's the Divine, and they will hear that voice long after I die.

Even so, I have particular hopes and longings. For example, I yearn to offer people a path to their own light and destiny. I want their experience of inspiration to last more than a few hours of chanting with me on some random Friday night. I desire that they feel the presence of a light fifty million times more powerful and that they sustain that divine connection for their entire life! Do you know what I mean? Can you feel this longing within me? This is what prompted this book.

So let's talk about you again.

You may wonder how you can make time for this practice. How can you possibly integrate something like this into your life with your responsibilities of family and work? I know from personal experience: it's a challenge. It doesn't matter who you are or how you cut it.

However, something magical happens when you prioritize practice; everything flows—life, work, family, everything. You can find a way through anything because staying spiritually connected makes you lighter, more able to stand up for yourself, more able to speak your truth, and more in tune with the cosmic energy of the Universe, the origin of all love and innovation. Any good idea in my life has come from this practice of Sādhanā, this daily tapping into the Infinity of my original light, my higher consciousness, and the flow of the Universe that loves me and everything in it.

This manual includes all five stages of the entire practice. In this chapter I include ways to start even if you do not have the full two and a half hours. Sometimes we just have to begin somewhere; even committing to thirty minutes a day will shift your life dramatically because now you are in connection with your original light.

The mind works so hard to serve us; it can do anything. And in its innocent effort to steer the ship, it tries hard to remain in control. This effort is futile, of course, because the flow of everyday life—not to mention the flow of Spirit—remains beyond the mind's control. And so frantic, incessant thoughts take over, as the mind increases its struggle. As yogīs, we understand and value the mind and its gifts, yet in order for us to commune with the Creator, to commune with our Divine Self, the mind must learn to attain stillness and quiet and experience positive vibration for at least some portion of the day. This is where regular practice comes in: establishing a connective pattern comforts the mind on the deepest of levels. Just as the sound of a mother's heartbeat comforts a crying infant, so too does spiritual practice soothe the ever-anxious mind. Essentially, you communicate to the mind that the way of soul, the way of Spirit, offers far more gratification and security than the mind's normal controlling patterns can bring. This message shifts everything; it's a complete paradigm shift for your entire life.

IDEAS TO BEGIN YOUR JOURNEY

The following practice ideas may take anywhere between thirty and ninety minutes. Actually, when we just start out, it can help us more to engage in shorter practices than, say, the entire Sādhanā as outlined in this book. Experiencing success in our psyches after incorporating a regular practice that is manageable is by far more important than a long and perfect practice. Think of these suggestions as building blocks that will eventually lead to your full practice. However, I highly recommend that you follow the instructions for stage one, "Preparing for the Aquarian Sādhanā," as given in chapter 4, while you work with the other stages and build up your practice. For your practice, especially when a Kundalini Yoga set is involved, please tune in with the Ādī Mantra, "ong namo gurū dayv namo," and end with "Long Time Sun." This will be a great way to intentionalize your practice.

- Recite Jap Jī either by yourself or with a partner. Please recite along with the companion CD; we purposefully recorded it slowly for people just learning the words. You can also take one Paurī of Jap Jī and recite it eleven times a day. Feel free to read Jap Jī in English, too.

- Experience and become comfortable with one of the Kundalini Yoga sets offered in appendix B.

- Chant the Aquarian Sādhanā Mantras with the *Light of the Naam with Long Ek Ong Kar* CD when you get up in the morning, cook breakfast, walk, jog, drive to work, or do any of your regular activities throughout the morning. You can even make up your own tunes and chant without music. By incorporating these chants into the beginning of your day, you infuse yourself and your environment with positive energy.

- Practice a Kundalini Yoga set first, and then sit still in a meditative posture and chant the Aquarian Sādhanā Mantras. Ideally one would practice all of the chants from start to finish as specified. If you do not have time to do all of the chants, please just do what you have time for. When we practice in a state of love, we please the Divine.

- Practice an element of the fifth stage (chapter 8). Bow to something greater than yourself in a Gurdwārā or any other place of worship, or build an altar with images and symbols that uplift you and inspire you to bow. You can also offer a daily prayer. I encourage you to stand up and speak to God—use the Sikh format of the Ardās, pray from your own tradition, or voice other words that resonate deeply with you. Finally, you can ask God to speak to you through a daily reading from a spiritual text. Surely, She or He will.

EXPERIENCING THE FULL SĀDHANĀ

Whatever you choose, I encourage you to find ways to build up to the full Sādhanā. Tune in to what works for your body, mind, and spirit, and start there. If the yoga postures work for you, you can start there as your first building block; add additional stages as you become more comfortable to finally reach the full practice. This process may take time, even years, and you will experience a natural ebb and flow based on the seasons, your health, and your karma. Additionally, it really helps to join with community and friends on a regular basis to practice; this will also help you build up to doing the entire Sādhanā. I recommend practicing with others at least once a week, if not more. I'll talk about the benefits of community practice more in the next chapter.

FORTY-, NINETY-, ONE-THOUSAND-DAY PRACTICE

I encourage you to pick one of the ideas mentioned above or do the entire Aquarian Sādhanā for a minimum of forty days. This period of time allows us to cycle through the human experience: We start off with a lot of enthusiasm. We get tested. We hit a wall. We pass the test. We scale the wall. We experience victory. Amazing! If I want to conquer any obstacle in my life, I pick a meditation and do it for forty days; without fail, the whole situation shifts, and I become healed. I kid you not; it works! But here's a crucial point: you must do it for yourself. You can't do it for your spouse or children. You can't do it for approval or applause. You simply have to do it for yourself. Remember: the forty-day period is key. Yogi Bhajan taught that after forty days of a practice, we break a bad habit; after ninety days, we create new patterns; after one thousand days, we attain mastery.[2]

I invite you to join us at Summer Solstice in Rām Dās Puri as two thousand people chant at the top of their lungs into the open desert sky. This is my heart's home. Many of these practitioners have done the Aquarian Sādhanā for longer than a thousand days; the experience of practicing with them is absolutely mind-blowingly beautiful. I know "mind-blowingly" is not a word, but for this occasion it just seems so perfect.

FOR THE LOVE OF IT

If you stick with this practice, three distinct stages will mark the road map of your experience: Sādhanā, Arādhanā, and Prabhupatī.[3]

The first, Sādhanā, refers to the practice itself. It includes finding a place to meditate, carving out time in your life, and actually getting yourself there. You can get yourself to the practice by multiple means. In this stage, take note of any "should" that comes up for you: I "should" sit down and practice, I "should" know this chant by now, I "should" be more comfortable with this posture, and so on. Wherever there is a "should," there is an equal and opposite "shouldn't," and soon you may find your mind talking you out of things you thought you should do just last week. None of this will help you very much and—as I mentioned before—neither will engaging the Sādhanā in order to get approval from others. You won't continue to practice if you succumb to these pitfalls. Instead, keep returning to the original longing of your soul; from this place, allow your practice to evolve and become a loving habit. You *must* have love—pure love—for yourself, as well as love for the practice. From this place of love, you can do the important work to heal yourself, clear your mind, and unload your subconscious. Doing all of this results in you becoming present in your life as the beautiful radiant soul-being that you are.

The next phase, Arādhanā, refers to connecting to the Universal Self. After you develop the habit, rising to the challenge of regular morning practice, the next step is to actually connect. We can easily end up disconnecting. That is, instead of allowing ourselves to descend into a state of thoughtlessness and universal consciousness, we remain in a surface-level awareness, concerned with our own needs and desires. In Arādhanā we allow ourselves to go deeper, and our meditation becomes real. As we travel beyond our individual consciousness into the expansive cosmic awareness, our subconscious gets cleared in ways that we could never imagine.

Finally, Prabhupati, which literally means Spouse of God, refers to one who has obtained mastery. In this phase, you experience sheer joy in the practice. You no longer have to put effort into getting up in the morning; your practice gets you up! Having cleared your subconscious and arrived at mastery, you now meditate for the world with compassion and love for all human beings.

You may experience all three stages of the practice to a degree, but mastery of each remains a long way away. Relax within the process; this system is far from linear. Like a labyrinth, even as the pathway takes you closer to the center, you may in fact need to go to the outer edges a few more times before actually reaching your destination.

REFLECTIONS

Every yogī, saint, and sage I know of had a Sādhanā. Take Mother Teresa, for example. She got up every morning and prayed to God until she heard His voice. At one point in her life, Mother Teresa and her Sisters lived in a war zone. One morning during her prayers, God told her to travel to a particular spot in the war zone in order to take care of the wounded people there. Without notice to either warring side, Mother Teresa left in haste with the Sisters. By some incredible miracle, the fighting from both sides stopped for a few hours in the very spot they went to. Mother Theresa and her Sisters did what they could to help the people there, and when they returned home to safety, the fighting started up again. This is but one example of Mother Teresa's Sādhanā, and her mastery.

What's yours?

~ *Chapter Ten* ~

BLESSINGS FOR FAMILY
AND COMMUNITY

ਕਬਹੁ ਸਾਧਸੰਗਤਿ ਇਹੁ ਪਾਵੈ ॥

kabahū sādhasangat ih(u) pāvai.

Sometimes, this being attains the company of the Holy.

ਉਸੁ ਅਸਥਾਨ ਤੇ ਬਹੁਰਿ ਨ ਆਵੈ ॥

ous asathān thay bahur na āvai.

From that place, he does not have to come back again.

ਅੰਤਰਿ ਹੋਇ ਗਿਆਨ ਪਰਗਾਸੁ ॥

antar ho-i giān paragās.

The light of spiritual wisdom dawns within.

ਉਸੁ ਅਸਥਾਨ ਕਾ ਨਹੀ ਬਿਨਾਸੁ ॥

ous asathān kā nahī binās.

That place does not perish.

GURŪ ARJAN, *SIRĪ GURŪ GRANTH SĀHIB JĪ*[1]

143

I feel so happy that I grew up in such a loving family and community in which I experienced the Aquarian Sādhanā. It helped me know without a doubt that children can experience God, meditation, and spiritual discipline in a loving and joyful way. I have come to appreciate how vital community is in the experience of this morning practice. In this chapter I will explore the blessings of family and community.

FAMILY LIFE IN THE AQUARIAN SĀDHANĀ

"Don't worry so much about giving your children cars.
Worry about giving them Samskaras!"
H. H. PUJYA SWAMI CHIDANAND SARASWATIJI[2]

Samskaras are the imprints left on the subconscious mind by experience in this life or previous lives; they color our entire life—our nature, responses, and states of mind. Samskaras are simply impressions on the psyche of the child, or any human being, created by the vibration of an experience: a conversation with a friend, a trip to the mall, or a family dinner. When we provide positive Samskaras for our children, we contribute to their overall capacity to live in the vibration of love and light and that becomes their foundation as adults. We can even do this before conception! The vibration and intention of the mother and father at the time of conception lay the foundation for the child—it all goes back to how the sperm approaches the egg. What is the relationship of the mother and father? What are the thoughts and feelings they have for each other? It all matters! Every single conversation with your beloved sets the tone for the environment of the child. And that is not to say that we can't have arguments. We just need a way to pass through life consciously: we strive to see, feel, and relate to the Divine within each other. For this reason, following a daily spiritual practice is incredibly important.

The vibration between a pregnant mother and the father of the child directly influences the beautiful soul in the mother's womb.[3] For the mother, practicing yoga and meditation will help lead to a blissful birth, but it will also improve the environment for that child's soul and body. Yogi Bhajan taught that, during pregnancy, the mother imparts most of what she will ever teach her child through vibrations, thoughts, and words. If the mother has not released the energy of childhood traumas and wounded relationships, she will face a lot of obstacles in giving the purity of her essential self and vibration to her child. So, the father has it pretty easy here, right? No way! The baby directly feels and understands the father's connection to himself and to the mother. Balanced vibrations between mother and father provide a sense of stability. The father's daily practice is just as important. And for people in same-sex marriages and relationships that include parenting, I believe these concepts still apply.

After childbirth, most of us experience the sheer overwhelm of parenthood, and we regularly find difficulty providing the best spiritual environment for our children. One mother told me that she had practiced the full Aquarian Sādhanā for many years, but then she had three sons, all two years apart, and her regular practice fell to pieces. In distress, she talked to Yogi Bhajan about it, and he comforted her by saying that being a good mother was now her Sādhanā. As a young mother, I took this story to heart. It helped me see that being a parent is a process, a job. I realized how important it is to remain in my Divinity to support my child and that this quest would be like nothing else I had experienced! I also understood that my spiritual practice was more important than anything and that I'd have to find ways to incorporate spirituality into my daily life even if I did not have the time to sit down and meditate. I could chant while I cooked or did the laundry and housecleaning. I could breathe deeply as I held my daughter. Suddenly, I realized how much time I had for spiritual practice! Anyone can have this perspective. Take a deep breath, take another deep breath, and repeat. When we breathe deeply, we realize that we have exactly the amount of time we are supposed to have.

Sādhanā remains one of the highest priorities for my husband and me. With our new baby daughter, Jap Preet, we had to experiment with how to integrate this practice into our new family. Sometimes we went to group Sādhanā; sometimes we practiced at home. By the time Jap Preet turned three, she knew what was happening and that it would happen almost every day. I feel confident that we provided our daughter with many positive Samskaras. She would often wake up briefly, eyes barely open, just listening to everyone chanting or watching the yoga postures unfold in the group practice, and then fall right back asleep. We did the Sādhanā in love and enjoyment, and in this space my daughter got to experience it in her own way.

When she got a little older, I attempted to get Jap Preet to practice "with" me. These attempts failed miserably, because my strong, fierce daughter could perceive any attempts on my part to control her. I feel incredibly grateful for her strong will because I have already seen how it serves her bright soul within. Yet I often wondered how in the world I was ever going to impart something that was so important to me. I would say, "Let's chant together!" That was regularly met by a vigorous "No," often accompanied by Jap Preet marching out of the room! I also tried, "Time to do our Sādhanā!" Yeah, right. She gave me her best "you've gotta be kidding me" look.

The answer came one day when one of my dear friends, whom my daughter loves very much, took Jap Preet onto her lap. At this time my daughter was five. I sat right next to her, engaged in conversation with someone else. My friend tickled Jap Preet, snuggled with her, and said, "You know, we all love your mama's tunes so much!" She and Jap Preet began chanting one of the Sādhanā tunes, "Rakhay Rakhanahār," which I chant every morning. Most mornings I thought my daughter was asleep during this chant, but she knew all the words and sang right along with my friend with a smile on her face. Take-home lesson for Mama: your daughter is learning more from your example than anything else at this point.

We can't coerce our children in most things, and this holds especially true for spiritual practice; we simply have to invite them into their own path. I'm not an expert in this area, but I can share something that truly helped support our family spiritual practice: community! When my family joins in with community practice, our daughter loves it. It makes all the difference for her to connect with and see other children.

Last year, my husband and I helped offer a Kundalini Yoga teacher training course in Peterborough, New Hampshire, our home at the time. As part of the course, we practiced the Aquarian Sādhanā. One morning, under the stars of an early morning sky, about fifty participants and staff quietly made their way to a large gym transformed into our beautiful teaching space by a touch of flowers and incense. Our daughter was cozy and asleep in her sleeping bag as we began our Jap Jī. Other parents came with their children as well, also bundled up in blankets. And then it happened.

Pop! Up went my daughter's head. And just in that moment her good friend, Amrit Atma, arrived with her mother. Amrit Atma looked sleepy, and I recognized her mother's body language—it resembled mine. It said, "Just stay quiet and calm, and maybe my daughter will go back to sleep."

"Is Amrit Atma here?" Jap Preet asked in a surprisingly awake tone.

I nodded my head yes, and pointed in the direction of her newly arrived friend, dutifully making the "shhhh" symbol, and knowing all too well that it would be ignored. Jap Preet skipped over to her friend, and the two girls embraced in a bear hug, chatting away. It was about four in the morning. Amrit Atma's mother and I exchanged surrendered smiles.

As the yoga began, the girls took part by performing some curious variation of the poses. Downward dog, followed by cobra, and then a sprinkling of skips accompanied with an uproar of giggles. Soon the other children woke up and joined this little celebration—it became a Sādhanā gang with the kids. I looked worriedly around the room, concerned that the other practitioners were being disturbed, but I only found smiling faces and even a few chuckles. Realizing that I was probably the most concerned person in the room, I took a deep breath and did the practice, sinking into a deep healing place as I realized how happy my daughter truly was. As the chants began, the girls ended up in the back of the gym, chanting together. Finally, as we all dove deeper into the etheric blue sounds of the chants, the children slowly made their way back to their parents and cuddled into their sleeping bags for a nap bathed in the Name.

Perhaps just as important as the opportunity to spiritually engage this way with community and other children is the presence of sweets. Never underestimate the power of sweets with children! In Gurdwārā, at the end of the fifth stage of the Aquarian Sādhanā, my daughter totally looks forward to sweet Gur Prasād. Yet, let me say that with the community practice and the touch of the Gurū, these sweets become the true delight, the Nectar that all of our souls long for.

Once there was a boy named Farid whose mother encouraged him to meditate every day by promising that God would leave him a treat under his meditation mat.[4] (Of course, Farid's mother taught him how to meditate with direct, simple, and true language—just as I recommend that all parents do.) Every day, while Farid meditated with his eyes closed, his mother placed some sweets under his mat. Farid would finish his meditation and immediately look under the mat, find the sweets, and delightfully eat them all. His mother did this for several days in a row until, one day, Farid finished his meditation and just sat with a blissful smile on his face—he was so happy and so peaceful. To his mother's surprise, Farid did not look under his mat for the sweets. She asked him curiously, "Why do you not wish to look for the sweets this morning?"

Farid replied, "Oh mother, when you have tasted the sweetness of the Holy Nām (the vibration of God's Name), there is nothing sweeter!"

That was a great victory for Farid's mother, and a potential victory for all parents: sharing the gift of Spirit with our children. We have to share; we have to at least make the effort. Remember that every saint, every sage, every enlightened being on this planet had a mother, and maybe both parents, to impart the gift of connecting to Spirit and Love. Yogi Bhajan taught us that Jesus first learned that he was the Son of God from his mother, Mary.[5] In a similar way, we also must impart this golden knowledge to our children, one way or another. In the moments when we are in our center, these are good times to talk to our children about the importance of a deep breath, chanting to uplift the mood, the interior "golden city" that we can explore when we close our eyes, the God that is all around us and in every being, along with the many more insights each of us have as parents. We have the capacity to be teachers for our children. As we work with them to brush their teeth and comb their hair on a day-to-day basis, we can also help them find ways to clear their energy.

Finally, I want to encourage you to have your children attend yoga classes and summer camps or schools that focus on spiritual growth. Peers and good teachers offer unique support that will additionally benefit your kids, fostering a natural joy to their spiritual practice. I have also listed some wonderful children's resources at the end of this manual, and I invite you to look into them if you feel interested.

BENEFITS OF COMMUNITY PRACTICE

"Doing Sādhanā in a group develops group consciousness. At the beginning of Sādhanā everyone has a different vibration. Some have traces of dreams, others are already filled with concerns for the day, and still others come with different expectations about Sādhanā. The more people there are, the more these individual differences balance out and create a harmony. The happiness of one person balances the sadness of another. Then the entire group finds its energy directed by the activity of the Sādhanā itself. The individual Auras merge and form a group Aura. When the group is well tuned to the Infinite, a rainbow Aura forms that reflects all colors; a bluish color of sincerity and devotion predominates. The auric transformation aids the practitioner in making the step beyond ego centeredness."

YOGI BHAJAN, *THE AQUARIAN TEACHER*[6]

In sharing this practice with people, I realize once again the vital role of community. Community brings answers, healing, and support in ways that nothing else can. You can certainly do the Aquarian Sādhanā at home by yourself and experience amazing effects, but I distinctly remember Yogi Bhajan teaching us that community practice is ten times more powerful. For this reason I make incredible efforts to participate with community as much as possible. Here are some of the key benefits to community practice:

- **Joining of Psyches.** If one person in the group goes very deep in their meditation, they without fail take everyone else with them. As we breathe together, practice yoga together, and chant together, we join our psyches. Likewise, if someone needs healing, the group energy will help.

- **Purification of the Self.** The guy in front of you decides to pass a little gas. Or perhaps the lady sitting to your right sings terribly off-key. Or someone keeps opening up the window right after you have closed it. If you are wondering whether I take these examples from personal experience, the answer is yes! I would even venture to say that I also annoy

my community members from time to time. If we can keep
our sense of humor, maintain our center, and roll with it,
so to speak, these types of frustrations become wonderful
opportunities to purify ourselves. When challenges arise
in the morning practice, they are amplified because we go
extremely deep within ourselves, no longer just existing on
the periphery. So as challenges arise, instead of falling into
habitual roles of victim or complainer, we look at them as
opportunities to breathe deeply and move through the lesson
currently presented to us. In this way, we become lighter,
freer, and more able to live in a way that reflects the spirit,
as opposed to only replaying our karmic lessons.

- **Transfer of Knowledge and Experience via Osmosis.**
  For beginners and seasoned meditators alike, group practice
  becomes an opportunity to share in experience. If someone
  has a pure experience of the teachings, everyone present
  receives some of it. The experience can be transferred to
  you by the teacher guiding the Sādhanā or even by someone
  sitting next to you who is following the instruction, perhaps
  even for the first time. For this reason, I highly recommend
  that if you want to master this practice, find a group that
  includes beginners and more seasoned practitioners who
  can share with you via this type of osmosis. By just sitting
  next to someone who has been steeped in Sādhanā for many
  years, we partake in a precious energetic imprint as we sense
  their straight spine, breath, and awareness. Likewise, those
  who have been around for a while have much to learn from
  beginners; the humility of learning for the first time creates
  a space for the purity of the soul to emerge.

- **Increased Capacity to Communicate.** After practicing
  together, communication flows at a deeper level. We
  simultaneously fulfill our own needs and goals as we
  help meet our neighbors' as well. In this way we serve
  one another through our practice. Magic happens when

communities practice together; after Sādhanā, people freely ask and offer assistance, all in the flow of joy and peace.

- **Selfless Service.** Through Seva, we have the opportunity to burn karma and perhaps more importantly to experience a level of abundance and joy unmatched on this planet. Open your doors to others, play the music for the Sādhanā, prepare a yummy breakfast . . . There are countless ways to provide in this way. The Aquarian Sādhanā is always offered free of charge.

CREATING SACRED COMMUNITY

So, let's say you want to create sacred community through the Aquarian Sādhanā. Please remember that, as I present it in this book, community can mean just you and a friend successfully supporting each other or it can look like a crowded room packed with enthusiastic practitioners. The main idea is that you weave a support system together, and the Aquarian Sādhanā works as an incredibly effective community support mechanism.

Continuity is key. Start off with something you know you can handle and stick with it. For example, if you know that you can offer the Aquarian Sādhanā out of your home or yoga center once a week on a regular basis, this will create a beneficial vibration that people can rely on. However, if you advertise a schedule but can't follow through, the dissonance created will leave others on shaky ground; if people show up to practice and you aren't there, they likely won't come back again.

We practiced a daily Aquarian Sādhanā in Eugene, Oregon, and put up fliers around town inviting people to join us. Six months after doing this, a woman joined us who had been looking at our flier; it was in the window of the restaurant where she worked and it took her six months to schedule a way to make it to the Sādhanā. She was so grateful to finally attend.

Community practice creates sacred space. If we look at every church, synagogue, mosque, temple, Gurdwārā, and other sacred gathering places on this planet, those that vibrate peace and sanctity always involve the presence of human hands and hearts, and they also welcome children. We build temples with stones and steel, but the real sweetness comes with our presence, our voices. People make a space what it is. It's funny: People often want to travel across the world to experience spirituality, as if it were a thing that existed somewhere outside of them. And yet, it only exists within. We are the ones who make our community spaces sacred or not.

Of course, we can admire certain locations and attempt to infuse our homes and communities with their gifts. As a Sikh, I look to the Golden Temple in Amritsar, India. Its doors are open to all. Sacred music plays from early morning to late at night every day. Whoever enters the Golden Temple can receive a free meal, and ten thousand people are served every day. So I try to find ways to apply that generosity to my own life. Can I offer the Aquarian Sādhanā to anyone who wants to attend? Do people attend whom I wouldn't normally hang out with? Or have I been trying to make my spiritual group into some kind of exclusive club? Contemplating in this way, we can act according to our heart's deepest wisdom and bring the Divine into our daily lives, building sacred spaces together as a community.

My mother's ashram offers Gurdwārā once a month on Sunday. The *Kirtan,* or sacred chanting, starts at around 10 a.m. and often goes until one in the afternoon. Afterward, the ashram serves a *Langar,* or a free community meal. For years, a guy named Tom has come in precisely when they serve the food; he shows up without fail! He doesn't spend time with people socially or engage in any type of spiritual practice with the community, but because he's a regular when it comes to mealtime, the ashram has embraced him as a beloved member.

RESOURCES FOR PRACTICING THE AQUARIAN SĀDHANĀ IN COMMUNITY

Let's say that community practice interests you, but you don't know where to begin. Check out these ideas, outlined in more detail in the resources section:

- Find a nearby Kundalini Yoga teacher who offers the Aquarian Sādhanā.

- Attend a festival that holds the Aquarian Sādhanā (for example, try the Sat Nam Fest gatherings sponsored by Spirit Voyage, or Summer and Winter Solstice hosted by 3HO).

- Become a certified Kundalini Yoga teacher. Get empowered to host the Aquarian Sādhanā and connect with others who practice it.

Whether you have the means to practice in physical community or not, I invite you to consciously reach out and feel all of us out there, thousands and thousands of us, from this practice and every practice from every walk of life. We all contribute to the energy of positivity, light, and truth on this planet. Through our practice, we become beacons of light.

EPILOGUE

We have reached the place where my words end and you begin. I love this Aquarian Sādhanā practice, and after writing this book I love it even more. I hope something in here has inspired you, or at least made you chuckle, or helped you begin your daily practice. After finishing this book the other morning, I was in my kitchen listening to a recording of Yogi Bhajan. When he said the following words, I stopped doing the dishes and just cried. The tears poured forth, as if the months and months of writing released themselves onto my countertop. They were not tears of sadness, but rather joy and humility, as I realized that my teacher was speaking to me in that moment of completion. My life and this book are a part of an incredible cosmic effort whose energy, purity, and miracle have been in place long before me, and will continue long after. I invite you to let these words of Yogi Bhajan speak to you as you begin your journey:

> "The path is already laid. Simply you are the first one to walk over it. We are all going together, with our egos, to the Age of Aquarius. That means your consciousness will guide you, and you will understand the meaning of what life is all about."[1]

God bless you.

With all the Love in my heart,
Snatam Kaur

ACKNOWLEDGMENTS

I am grateful to my husband, Sopurkh Singh, who is my Beloved, dear friend, and partner in meditating, teaching, and parenting. Through his dedication to the Aquarian Sādhanā, my practice has deepened, and we have been able to raise our daughter in the vibration of our spiritual path. I am so grateful for all of those mornings when he carried our young daughter through the snow, up and down mountain trails, and across other types of harsh terrain so that we could all engage in the Sadhānā and benefit together. Thank you to my daughter, Jap Preet Kaur, who keeps it real for me, always reminding me to be in my heart and showing me what true love is. I am grateful to Karan and Simranpreet of Spirit Voyage for supporting this vision and helping to bring it forth. To the wise and intelligent Sat Purkh Kaur Khalsa: you are a wonderful editor, and I am so blessed to have worked with you. My gratitude to Himmat Singh Khalsa for his loving support in helping me with my Jap Jī pronunciation and finding a good transliteration system. I also give thanks to Hari Kirin Kaur Khalsa for all of her wonderful advice and presence in this project. To my mother, Prabhu Nam Kaur, and stepfather, Sat Santokh Singh: thank you for all that you taught me through your incredible example of devotion and love on the spiritual path. My gratitude to Siri Sikhdar Sahiba Guru Amrit Kaur Khalsa, Guru Kirn Kaur Khalsa, and Siri Neel Kaur Khalsa of KRI for your wonderful insight that helped maintain the sanctity of the teachings presented here. I am grateful to all those who helped me to create such beautiful music for this book: Thomas Barquee, Ajeet Kaur, Siri Kirtan Kaur, Sukhmani Kaur, Gurusangat Singh, and others. And thank you to our communities in southern New Hampshire; Santa Cruz, California; Los Angeles, California; Eugene, Oregon; Española, New Mexico; and the entire global community of 3HO for giving me countless experiences of upliftment and grace that inspired this book.

JAP JĪ SĀHIB[1]

ਜਪੁ ਜੀ ਸਾਹਿਬ

Jap Jī Sāhib

Great Meditation and Recitation of the Soul

ੴ ਸਤਿਨਾਮੁ ਕਰਤਾ ਪੁਰਖੁ ਨਿਰਭਉ ਨਿਰਵੈਰੁ
ਅਕਾਲ ਮੂਰਤਿ ਅਜੂਨੀ ਸੈਭੰ ਗੁਰ ਪ੍ਰਸਾਦਿ ॥

ek ong kār satinām karatā purakh nirabha-u niravair
akāl mūrat ajūnī saibhang gur prasād.

*One Universal Creator God. The Name Is Truth. Creative Being Personified.
No Fear. No Hatred. Image of The Undying, Beyond Birth, Self-Existent.
By Gurū's Grace ~*

॥ ਜਪੁ ॥

jap.

Chant and Meditate:

ਆਦਿ ਸਚੁ ਜੁਗਾਦਿ ਸਚੁ ॥

ād sach jugād sach.

True in the Primal Beginning. True throughout the Ages.

ਹੈ ਭੀ ਸਚੁ ਨਾਨਕ ਹੋਸੀ ਭੀ ਸਚੁ ॥੧॥

hai bhī sach nānak hosī bhī sach. ॥ 1॥

True Here and Now. O Nānak, Forever and Ever True. ‖ 1‖

ਸੋਚੈ ਸੋਚਿ ਨ ਹੋਵਈ ਜੇ ਸੋਚੀ ਲਖ ਵਾਰ ॥

sochai soch na hova-ī jay sochī lakh vār.

By thinking, He cannot be reduced to thought,
even by thinking hundreds of thousands of times.

ਚੁਪੈ ਚੁਪ ਨ ਹੋਵਈ ਜੇ ਲਾਇ ਰਹਾ ਲਿਵ ਤਾਰ ॥

chupai chup na hova-ī jay lā-i rahā liv tār.

By remaining silent, inner silence is not obtained,
even by remaining lovingly absorbed deep within.

ਭੁਖਿਆ ਭੁਖ ਨ ਉਤਰੀ ਜੇ ਬੰਨਾ ਪੁਰੀਆ ਭਾਰ ॥

bhukhi-ā bhukh na utarī jay banā purī-ā bhār.

The hunger of the hungry is not appeased,
even by piling up loads of worldly goods.

ਸਹਸ ਸਿਆਣਪਾ ਲਖ ਹੋਹਿ ਤ ਇਕ ਨ ਚਲੈ ਨਾਲਿ ॥

sahas si-āṉapā lakh hoh(i) ta ik na chalai nāl.

Hundreds of thousands of clever tricks, but not even one of them
will go along with you in the end.

ਕਿਵ ਸਚਿਆਰਾ ਹੋਈਐ ਕਿਵ ਕੂੜੈ ਤੁਟੈ ਪਾਲਿ ॥

kiv sachi-ārā ho-ī-ai kiv kūṟai tuṯai pāl.

So how can you become truthful? And how can the veil of illusion be torn away?

ਹੁਕਮਿ ਰਜਾਈ ਚਲਣਾ ਨਾਨਕ ਲਿਖਿਆ ਨਾਲਿ ॥੧॥

hukam rajā-ī chalaṉā nānak likhi-ā nāl. ॥ 1॥

O Nānak, it is written that you shall obey the Hukam of His Command,
and walk in the Way of His Will. ॥ 1॥

ਹੁਕਮੀ ਹੋਵਨਿ ਆਕਾਰ ਹੁਕਮੁ ਨ ਕਹਿਆ ਜਾਈ ॥

hukamī hovan ākār hukam na kahi-ā jā-ī.

By His Command, bodies are created; His Command cannot be described.

ਹੁਕਮੀ ਹੋਵਨਿ ਜੀਅ ਹੁਕਮਿ ਮਿਲੈ ਵਡਿਆਈ ॥

hukamī hovan jī-a hukam milai vadi-ā-ī.

By His Command, souls come into being; by His Command,
glory and greatness are obtained.

ਹੁਕਮੀ ਉਤਮੁ ਨੀਚੁ ਹੁਕਮਿ ਲਿਖਿ ਦੁਖ ਸੁਖ ਪਾਈਅਹਿ ॥

hukamī utam nīch hukam likh dukh sukh pā-ī-a-h(i).

By His Command, some are high and some are low; by His Written Command,
pain and pleasure are obtained.

ਇਕਨਾ ਹੁਕਮੀ ਬਖਸੀਸ ਇਕਿ ਹੁਕਮੀ ਸਦਾ ਭਵਾਈਅਹਿ ॥

ikanā hukamī bakhasīs ik hukamī sadā bhavā-ī-a-h(i).

Some, by His Command, are blessed and forgiven; others, by His Command,
wander aimlessly forever.

ਹੁਕਮੈ ਅੰਦਰਿ ਸਭੁ ਕੋ ਬਾਹਰਿ ਹੁਕਮ ਨ ਕੋਇ ॥

hukamai andar sabh ko bāhar hukam na ko-i.

Everyone is subject to His Command; no one is beyond His Command.

ਨਾਨਕ ਹੁਕਮੈ ਜੇ ਬੁਝੈ ਤ ਹਉਮੈ ਕਹੈ ਨ ਕੋਇ ॥੨॥

nānak hukamai jay bujhai ta ha-umai kahai na ko-i. || 2||

O Nānak, one who understands His Command, does not speak in ego. ||2||

ਗਾਵੈ ਕੋ ਤਾਣੁ ਹੋਵੈ ਕਿਸੈ ਤਾਣੁ ॥

gāvai ko tāṇ hovai kisai tāṇ.

Some sing of His Power—who has that Power?

ਗਾਵੈ ਕੋ ਦਾਤਿ ਜਾਣੈ ਨੀਸਾਣੁ ॥

gāvai ko dāt jāṇai nīsāṇ.

Some sing of His Gifts, and know His Sign and Insignia.

ਗਾਵੈ ਕੋ ਗੁਣ ਵਡਿਆਈਆ ਚਾਰ ॥

gāvai ko guṇ vaḍi-ā-ī-ā chār.

Some sing of His Glorious Virtues, Greatness, and Beauty.

ਗਾਵੈ ਕੋ ਵਿਦਿਆ ਵਿਖਮੁ ਵੀਚਾਰੁ ॥

gāvai ko vidi-ā vikham vīchār.

Some sing of knowledge obtained of Him, through difficult philosophical studies.

ਗਾਵੈ ਕੋ ਸਾਜਿ ਕਰੇ ਤਨੁ ਖੇਹ ॥

gāvai ko sāj karay tan khayh.

Some sing that He fashions the body, and then again reduces it to dust.

ਗਾਵੈ ਕੋ ਜੀਅ ਲੈ ਫਿਰਿ ਦੇਹ ॥

gāvai ko jī-a lai phir dayh.

Some sing that He takes life away, and then again restores it.

ਗਾਵੈ ਕੋ ਜਾਪੈ ਦਿਸੈ ਦੂਰਿ ॥

gāvai ko jāpai disai dūr.

Some sing that He seems so very far away.

ਗਾਵੈ ਕੋ ਵੇਖੈ ਹਾਦਰਾ ਹਦੂਰਿ ॥

gāvai ko vaykhai hādarā hadūr.

Some sing that He watches over us, face to face, ever-present.

ਕਥਨਾ ਕਥੀ ਨ ਆਵੈ ਤੋਟਿ ॥

kathanā kathī na āvai toṭ.

There is no shortage of those who preach and teach.

ਕਥਿ ਕਥਿ ਕਥੀ ਕੋਟੀ ਕੋਟਿ ਕੋਟਿ ॥

kath kath kathī koṭī koṭ koṭ.

Millions upon millions offer millions of sermons and stories.

ਦੇਦਾ ਦੇ ਲੈਦੇ ਥਕਿ ਪਾਹਿ ॥

daydā day laiday thak pāh(i).

The Great Giver keeps on giving, while those who receive grow weary of receiving.

ਜੁਗਾ ਜੁਗੰਤਰਿ ਖਾਹੀ ਖਾਹਿ ॥

jugā jugantar khāhī khāh(i).

Throughout the ages, consumers consume.

ਹੁਕਮੀ ਹੁਕਮੁ ਚਲਾਏ ਰਾਹੁ ॥

hukamī hukam chalā-ay rāh(u).

The Commander, by His Command, leads us to walk on the Path.

ਨਾਨਕ ਵਿਗਸੈ ਵੇਪਰਵਾਹੁ ॥੩॥

nānak vigasai vayparavāh(u). || 3||

O Nānak, He blossoms forth, Carefree and Untroubled. ||3||

ਸਾਚਾ ਸਾਹਿਬੁ ਸਾਚੁ ਨਾਇ ਭਾਖਿਆ ਭਾਉ ਅਪਾਰੁ ॥

sāchā sāhib sāch nā-i bhākhi-ā bhā-u apār.

True is the Master, True is His Name—speak it with infinite love.

ਆਖਹਿ ਮੰਗਹਿ ਦੇਹਿ ਦੇਹਿ ਦਾਤਿ ਕਰੇ ਦਾਤਾਰੁ ॥

ākhah(i) mangah(i) dayh(i) dayh(i) dāt karay dātār.

People beg and pray, "Give to us, give to us," and the Great Giver gives His Gifts.

ਫੇਰਿ ਕਿ ਅਗੈ ਰਖੀਐ ਜਿਤੁ ਦਿਸੈ ਦਰਬਾਰੁ ॥

phayr ki agai rakhī-ai jit disai darabār.

So what offering can we place before Him,
by which we might see the Darabār of His Court?

ਮੁਹੌ ਕਿ ਬੋਲਣੁ ਬੋਲੀਐ ਜਿਤੁ ਸੁਣਿ ਧਰੇ ਪਿਆਰੁ ॥

muhau ki bolan bolī-ai jit sun dharay pi-ār.

What words can we speak to evoke His Love?

163

ਅੰਮ੍ਰਿਤ ਵੇਲਾ ਸਚੁ ਨਾਉ ਵਡਿਆਈ ਵੀਚਾਰੁ ॥

amrit vaylā sach nā-u vaḏi-ā-ī vīchār.

In the Amrit Vaylā, the ambrosial hours before dawn, chant the True Name,
and contemplate His Glorious Greatness.

ਕਰਮੀ ਆਵੈ ਕਪੜਾ ਨਦਰੀ ਮੋਖੁ ਦੁਆਰੁ ॥

karamī āvai kapaṟā nadarī mokh du-ār.

By the karma of past actions, the robe of this physical body is obtained.
By His Grace, the Gate of Liberation is found.

ਨਾਨਕ ਏਵੈ ਜਾਣੀਐ ਸਭੁ ਆਪੇ ਸਚਿਆਰੁ ॥੪॥

nānak ayvai jāṉī-ai sabh āpay sachiār. || 4||

O Nānak, know this well: the True One Himself is All. || 4||

ਥਾਪਿਆ ਨ ਜਾਇ ਕੀਤਾ ਨ ਹੋਇ ॥

thāpi-ā na jā-i kītā na ho-i.

He cannot be established, He cannot be created.

ਆਪੇ ਆਪਿ ਨਿਰੰਜਨੁ ਸੋਇ ॥

āpay āp niranjan so-i.

He Himself is Immaculate and Pure.

ਜਿਨਿ ਸੇਵਿਆ ਤਿਨਿ ਪਾਇਆ ਮਾਨੁ ॥

jin sayvi-ā tin pā-i-ā mān.

Those who serve Him are honored.

ਨਾਨਕ ਗਾਵੀਐ ਗੁਣੀ ਨਿਧਾਨੁ ॥

nānak gāvī-ai guṉī nidhān.

O Nānak, sing of the Lord, the Treasure of Excellence.

ਗਾਵੀਐ ਸੁਣੀਐ ਮਨਿ ਰਖੀਐ ਭਾਉ ॥

gāvī-ai suṇī-ai man rakhī-ai bhā-u.

Sing, and listen, and let your mind be filled with love.

ਦੁਖੁ ਪਰਹਰਿ ਸੁਖੁ ਘਰਿ ਲੈ ਜਾਇ ॥

dukh parahar sukh ghar lai jā-i.

Having given up sorrow to God, take peace and go home with it.

ਗੁਰਮੁਖਿ ਨਾਦੰ ਗੁਰਮੁਖਿ ਵੇਦੰ ਗੁਰਮੁਖਿ ਰਹਿਆ ਸਮਾਈ ॥

guramukh nādang guramukh vaydang guramukh rahi-ā samā-ī.

The Gurū's Word is the Sound Current of the Naad; the Gurū's Word is the Wisdom of the Vedas; the Gurū's Word is all-pervading.

ਗੁਰੁ ਈਸਰੁ ਗੁਰੁ ਗੋਰਖੁ ਬਰਮਾ ਗੁਰੁ ਪਾਰਬਤੀ ਮਾਈ ॥

gur īsar gur gorakh baramā gur pārabatī mā-ī.

The Gurū is Shiva, the Gurū is Vishnu and Brahma; the Gurū is Pārvatī and Lakhshmī.

ਜੇ ਹਉ ਜਾਣਾ ਆਖਾ ਨਾਹੀ ਕਹਣਾ ਕਥਨੁ ਨ ਜਾਈ ॥

jay ha-u jāṇā ākhā nāhī kahaṇā kathan na jā-ī.

Even knowing God, I cannot describe Him; He cannot be described in words.

ਗੁਰਾ ਇਕ ਦੇਹਿ ਬੁਝਾਈ ॥

gurā ik dayh(i) bujhā-ī.

The Gurū has given me this one understanding:

ਸਭਨਾ ਜੀਆ ਕਾ ਇਕੁ ਦਾਤਾ ਸੋ ਮੈ ਵਿਸਰਿ ਨ ਜਾਈ ॥੫॥

sabhanā jī-ā kā ik dātā so mai visar na jā-ī. || 5||

there is only the One, the Giver of all souls. May I never forget Him! || 5||

ਤੀਰਥਿ ਨਾਵਾ ਜੇ ਤਿਸੁ ਭਾਵਾ ਵਿਣੁ ਭਾਣੇ ਕਿ ਨਾਇ ਕਰੀ ॥

tīrath nāvā jay tis bhāvā viṇ bhāṇay ki nā-i karī.

If I am pleasing to Him, then that is my pilgrimage and cleansing bath.
Without pleasing Him, what good are ritual cleansings?

ਜੇਤੀ ਸਿਰਠਿ ਉਪਾਈ ਵੇਖਾ ਵਿਣੁ ਕਰਮਾ ਕਿ ਮਿਲੈ ਲਈ ॥

jaytī siraṭh upā-ī vaykhā viṇ karamā ki milai la-ī.

I gaze upon all the created beings: without the karma of good actions,
what are they given to receive?

ਮਤਿ ਵਿਚਿ ਰਤਨ ਜਵਾਹਰ ਮਾਣਿਕ ਜੇ ਇਕ ਗੁਰ ਕੀ ਸਿਖ ਸੁਣੀ ॥

mat vich ratan javāhar māṇik jay ik gur kī sikh suṇī.

Within the mind are gems, jewels, and rubies,
if you listen to the Gurū's Teachings, even once.

ਗੁਰਾ ਇਕ ਦੇਹਿ ਬੁਝਾਈ ॥

gurā ik dayh(i) bujhā-ī.

The Gurū has given me this one understanding:

ਸਭਨਾ ਜੀਆ ਕਾ ਇਕੁ ਦਾਤਾ ਸੋ ਮੈ ਵਿਸਰਿ ਨ ਜਾਈ ॥੬॥

sabhanā jī-ā kā ik dātā so mai visar na jā-ī. || 6||

there is only the One, the Giver of all souls. May I never forget Him! || 6||

ਜੇ ਜੁਗ ਚਾਰੇ ਆਰਜਾ ਹੋਰ ਦਸੂਣੀ ਹੋਇ ॥

jay jug chāray ārajā hor dasūṇī ho-i.

Even if you could live throughout the four ages, or even ten times more,

ਨਵਾ ਖੰਡਾ ਵਿਚਿ ਜਾਣੀਐ ਨਾਲਿ ਚਲੈ ਸਭੁ ਕੋਇ ॥

navā khanḍā vich jāṇī-ai nāl chalai sabh ko-i.

and even if you were known throughout the nine continents and followed by all,

ਚੰਗਾ ਨਾਉ ਰਖਾਇ ਕੈ ਜਸੁ ਕੀਰਤਿ ਜਗਿ ਲੇਇ ॥

changā nā-u rakhā-i kai jas kīrat jag lay-i.

with a good name and reputation, with praise and fame throughout the world—

ਜੇ ਤਿਸੁ ਨਦਰਿ ਨ ਆਵਈ ਤ ਵਾਤ ਨ ਪੁਛੈ ਕੇ ॥

jay tis nadar na āva-ī ta vāt na puchhai kay.

*still, if the Lord does not bless you with His Glance of Grace, then who cares?
What is the use?*

ਕੀਟਾ ਅੰਦਰਿ ਕੀਟੁ ਕਰਿ ਦੋਸੀ ਦੋਸੁ ਧਰੇ ॥

kītā andar kīt kar dosī dos dharay.

*Among worms, you would be considered a lowly worm,
and even contemptible sinners would hold you in contempt.*

ਨਾਨਕ ਨਿਰਗੁਣਿ ਗੁਣੁ ਕਰੇ ਗੁਣਵੰਤਿਆ ਗੁਣੁ ਦੇ ॥

nānak niragun gun karay gunavanti-ā gun day.

*O Nānak, God blesses the unworthy with virtue, and bestows virtue on the
virtuous.*

ਤੇਹਾ ਕੋਇ ਨ ਸੁਝਈ ਜਿ ਤਿਸੁ ਗੁਣੁ ਕੋਇ ਕਰੇ ॥੭॥

tayhā ko-i na sujha-ī ji tis gun ko-i karay. ‖ 7‖

No one can even imagine anyone who can bestow virtue upon Him. ‖ 7‖

ਸੁਣਿਐ ਸਿਧ ਪੀਰ ਸੁਰਿ ਨਾਥ ॥

suni-ai sidh pīr sur nāth.

Listening—the Siddhas, the spiritual teachers, the heroic warriors, the yogic masters.

ਸੁਣਿਐ ਧਰਤਿ ਧਵਲ ਆਕਾਸ ॥

suni-ai dharat dhaval ākās.

Listening—the earth, its support and the Akāshic ethers.

ਸੁਣਿਐ ਦੀਪ ਲੋਅ ਪਾਤਾਲ ॥

suṇi-ai dīp lo-a pātāl.

*Listening—the oceans, the lands of the world,
and the nether regions of the underworld.*

ਸੁਣਿਐ ਪੋਹਿ ਨ ਸਕੈ ਕਾਲੁ ॥

suṇi-ai poh(i) na sakai kāl.

Listening—Death cannot even touch you.

ਨਾਨਕ ਭਗਤਾ ਸਦਾ ਵਿਗਾਸੁ ॥

nānak bhagatā sadā vigās.

O Nānak, the devotees are forever in bliss.

ਸੁਣਿਐ ਦੂਖ ਪਾਪ ਕਾ ਨਾਸੁ ॥੮॥

suṇi-ai dūkh pāp kā nās. || 8||

Listening—pain and sin are erased. || 8||

ਸੁਣਿਐ ਈਸਰੁ ਬਰਮਾ ਇੰਦੁ ॥

suṇi-ai īsar baramā ind.

Listening—Shiva, Brahma, and Indra.

ਸੁਣਿਐ ਮੁਖਿ ਸਾਲਾਹਣ ਮੰਦੁ ॥

suṇi-ai mukh sālāhaṉ mand.

Listening—even foul-mouthed people praise Him.

ਸੁਣਿਐ ਜੋਗ ਜੁਗਤਿ ਤਨਿ ਭੇਦ ॥

suṇi-ai jog jugat tan bhayd.

Listening—the technology of Yoga and the secrets of the body.

ਸੁਣਿਐ ਸਾਸਤ ਸਿਮ੍ਰਿਤਿ ਵੇਦ ॥

suṇi-ai sāsat simrit vayd.

Listening—the Shāstras, the Simritīs, and the Vedas.

ਨਾਨਕ ਭਗਤਾ ਸਦਾ ਵਿਗਾਸੁ ॥

nānak bhagatā sadā vigās.

O Nānak, the devotees are forever in bliss.

ਸੁਣਿਐ ਦੂਖ ਪਾਪ ਕਾ ਨਾਸੁ ॥੯॥

suṇi-ai dūkh pāp kā nās. || 9||

Listening—pain and sin are erased. || 9||

ਸੁਣਿਐ ਸਤੁ ਸੰਤੋਖੁ ਗਿਆਨੁ ॥

suṇi-ai sat santokh gi-ān.

Listening—truth, contentment, and spiritual wisdom.

ਸੁਣਿਐ ਅਠਸਠਿ ਕਾ ਇਸਨਾਨੁ ॥

suṇi-ai aṭhasaṭh kā isanān.

Listening—take your cleansing bath at the sixty-eight places of pilgrimage.

ਸੁਣਿਐ ਪੜਿ ਪੜਿ ਪਾਵਹਿ ਮਾਨੁ ॥

suṇi-ai paṛ paṛ pāvah(i) mān.

Listening—reading and reciting, honor is obtained.

ਸੁਣਿਐ ਲਾਗੈ ਸਹਜਿ ਧਿਆਨੁ ॥

suṇi-ai lāgai sahaj dhi-ān.

Listening—intuitively grasp the essence of meditation.

ਨਾਨਕ ਭਗਤਾ ਸਦਾ ਵਿਗਾਸੁ ॥

nānak bhagatā sadā vigās.

O Nānak, the devotees are forever in bliss.

ਸੁਣਿਐ ਦੂਖ ਪਾਪ ਕਾ ਨਾਸੁ ॥੧੦॥

suṇi-ai dūkh pāp kā nās. || 10||

Listening—pain and sin are erased. || 10||

ਸੁਣਿਐ ਸਰਾ ਗੁਣਾ ਕੇ ਗਾਹ ॥

suṇi-ai sarā guṇā kay gāh.

Listening—dive deep into the ocean of virtue.

ਸੁਣਿਐ ਸੇਖ ਪੀਰ ਪਾਤਿਸਾਹ ॥

suṇi-ai saykh pīr pātisāh.

Listening—the Sheiks, religious scholars, spiritual teachers, and emperors.

ਸੁਣਿਐ ਅੰਧੇ ਪਾਵਹਿ ਰਾਹੁ ॥

suṇi-ai andhay pāvah(i) rāh(u).

Listening—even the blind find the Path.

ਸੁਣਿਐ ਹਾਥ ਹੋਵੈ ਅਸਗਾਹੁ ॥

suṇi-ai hāth hovai asagāh(u).

Listening—the Unreachable comes within your grasp.

ਨਾਨਕ ਭਗਤਾ ਸਦਾ ਵਿਗਾਸੁ ॥

nānak bhagatā sadā vigās.

O Nānak, the devotees are forever in bliss.

ਸੁਣਿਐ ਦੂਖ ਪਾਪ ਕਾ ਨਾਸੁ ॥੧੧॥

suṇi-ai dūkh pāp kā nās. || 11||

Listening—pain and sin are erased. ||11||

ਮੰਨੇ ਕੀ ਗਤਿ ਕਹੀ ਨ ਜਾਇ ॥

manay kī gat kahī na jā-i.

The state of the faithful cannot be described.

ਜੇ ਕੋ ਕਹੈ ਪਿਛੈ ਪਛੁਤਾਇ ॥

jay ko kahai pichhai pachhutā-i.

One who tries to describe this shall regret the attempt.

ਕਾਗਦਿ ਕਲਮ ਨ ਲਿਖਣਹਾਰੁ ॥

kāgad kalam na likhaṇahār.

No paper, no pen, no scribe

ਮੰਨੇ ਕਾ ਬਹਿ ਕਰਨਿ ਵੀਚਾਰੁ ॥

manay kā bah(i) karan vīchār.

can record the state of the faithful.

ਐਸਾ ਨਾਮੁ ਨਿਰੰਜਨੁ ਹੋਇ ॥

aisā nām niranjan ho-i.

Such is the Name of the Immaculate Lord.

ਜੇ ਕੋ ਮੰਨਿ ਜਾਣੈ ਮਨਿ ਕੋਇ ॥੧੨॥

jay ko man jāṇai man ko-i. || 12||

Only one who has faith comes to know such a state of mind. || 12||

ਮੰਨੈ ਸੁਰਤਿ ਹੋਵੈ ਮਨਿ ਬੁਧਿ ॥

manai surat hovai man budh.

The faithful have intuitive awareness and intelligence.

ਮੰਨੈ ਸਗਲ ਭਵਣ ਕੀ ਸੁਧਿ ॥

manai sagal bhavaṇ kī sudh.

The faithful know about all worlds and realms.

ਮੰਨੈ ਮੁਹਿ ਚੋਟਾ ਨਾ ਖਾਇ ॥

manai muh(i) choṭā nā khā-i.

The faithful shall never be struck across the face.

ਮੰਨੈ ਜਮ ਕੈ ਸਾਥਿ ਨ ਜਾਇ ॥

manai jam kai sāth na jā-i.

The faithful do not have to go with the Messenger of Death.

ਐਸਾ ਨਾਮੁ ਨਿਰੰਜਨੁ ਹੋਇ ॥

aisā nām niranjan ho-i.

Such is the Name of the Immaculate Lord.

ਜੇ ਕੋ ਮੰਨਿ ਜਾਣੈ ਮਨਿ ਕੋਇ ॥੧੩॥

jay ko man jāṇai man ko-i. ‖ 13‖

Only one who has faith comes to know such a state of mind. ‖ 13‖

ਮੰਨੈ ਮਾਰਗਿ ਠਾਕ ਨ ਪਾਇ ॥

manai mārag ṭhāk na pā-i.

The path of the faithful shall never be blocked.

ਮੰਨੈ ਪਤਿ ਸਿਉ ਪਰਗਟੁ ਜਾਇ ॥

manai pat si-u paragaṭ jā-i.

The faithful shall depart with honor and fame.

ਮੰਨੈ ਮਗੁ ਨ ਚਲੈ ਪੰਥੁ ॥

manai mag na chalai panth.

The faithful do not follow empty religious rituals.

ਮੰਨੈ ਧਰਮ ਸੇਤੀ ਸਨਬੰਧੁ ॥

manai dharam saytī sanabandh.

The faithful are firmly bound to the Dharma.

ਐਸਾ ਨਾਮੁ ਨਿਰੰਜਨੁ ਹੋਇ ॥

aisā nām niranjan ho-i.

Such is the Name of the Immaculate Lord.

ਜੇ ਕੋ ਮੰਨਿ ਜਾਣੈ ਮਨਿ ਕੋਇ ॥੧੪॥

jay ko man jāṇai man ko-i. ‖ 14‖

Only one who has faith comes to know such a state of mind. ‖ 14‖

ਮੰਨੈ ਪਾਵਹਿ ਮੋਖੁ ਦੁਆਰੁ ॥

manai pāvah(i) mokh du-ār.

The faithful find the Door of Liberation.

ਮੰਨੈ ਪਰਵਾਰੈ ਸਾਧਾਰੁ ॥

manai paravārai sādhār.

The faithful uplift and redeem their family and relations.

ਮੰਨੈ ਤਰੈ ਤਾਰੇ ਗੁਰੁ ਸਿਖ ॥

manai tarai tāray gur sikh.

The faithful are saved and carried across with the Sikhs of the Gurū.

ਮੰਨੈ ਨਾਨਕ ਭਵਹਿ ਨ ਭਿਖ ॥

manai nānak bhavah(i) na bhikh.

The faithful, O Nānak, do not wander around begging.

ਐਸਾ ਨਾਮੁ ਨਿਰੰਜਨੁ ਹੋਇ ॥

aisā nām niranjan ho-i.

Such is the Name of the Immaculate Lord.

ਜੇ ਕੋ ਮੰਨਿ ਜਾਣੈ ਮਨਿ ਕੋਇ ॥੧੫॥

jay ko man jāṉai man ko-i. || 15||

Only one who has faith comes to know such a state of mind. || 15||

ਪੰਚ ਪਰਵਾਣ ਪੰਚ ਪਰਧਾਨੁ ॥

panch paravāṉ panch paradhān.

The chosen ones, the self-elect, are accepted and approved.

ਪੰਚੇ ਪਾਵਹਿ ਦਰਗਹਿ ਮਾਨੁ ॥

panchay pāvah(i) daragah(i) mān.

The chosen ones are honored in the Court of the Lord.

173

ਪੰਚੇ ਸੋਹਹਿ ਦਰਿ ਰਾਜਾਨੁ ॥

panchay sohah(i) dar rājān.

The chosen ones look beautiful in the courts of kings.

ਪੰਚਾ ਕਾ ਗੁਰੁ ਏਕੁ ਧਿਆਨੁ ॥

panchā kā gur ayk dhi-ān.

The chosen ones meditate single-mindedly on the Gurū.

ਜੇ ਕੋ ਕਹੈ ਕਰੈ ਵੀਚਾਰੁ ॥

jay ko kahai karai vīchār.

No matter how much anyone tries to explain and describe them,

ਕਰਤੇ ਕੈ ਕਰਣੈ ਨਾਹੀ ਸੁਮਾਰੁ ॥

karatay kai karaṇai nāhī sumār.

the actions of the Creator cannot be counted.

ਧੌਲੁ ਧਰਮੁ ਦਇਆ ਕਾ ਪੂਤੁ ॥

dhaul dharam da-i-ā kā pūt.

The mythical bull is Dharma, the son of compassion;

ਸੰਤੋਖੁ ਥਾਪਿ ਰਖਿਆ ਜਿਨਿ ਸੂਤਿ ॥

santokh thāp rakhi-ā jin sūt.

this is what patiently holds the Earth in its place.

ਜੇ ਕੋ ਬੁਝੈ ਹੋਵੈ ਸਚਿਆਰੁ ॥

jay ko bujhai hovai sachi-ār.

One who understands this becomes truthful.

ਧਵਲੈ ਉਪਰਿ ਕੇਤਾ ਭਾਰੁ ॥

dhavalai upar kaytā bhār.

What a great load there is on the bull!

174

ਧਰਤੀ ਹੋਰੁ ਪਰੈ ਹੋਰੁ ਹੋਰੁ ॥

dharatī hor parai hor hor.

So many worlds beyond this world—so very many!

ਤਿਸ ਤੇ ਭਾਰੁ ਤਲੈ ਕਵਣੁ ਜੋਰੁ ॥

tis tay bhār talai kavan jor.

What power holds them, and supports their weight?

ਜੀਅ ਜਾਤਿ ਰੰਗਾ ਕੇ ਨਾਵ ॥

jī-a jāt rangā kay nāv.

The names and the colors of the assorted species of beings

ਸਭਨਾ ਲਿਖਿਆ ਵੁੜੀ ਕਲਾਮ ॥

sabhanā likhi-ā vuṛī kalām.

were all inscribed by the Ever-flowing Pen of God.

ਏਹੁ ਲੇਖਾ ਲਿਖਿ ਜਾਣੈ ਕੋਇ ॥

ayh(u) laykhā likh jāṇai ko-i.

Who knows how to write this account?

ਲੇਖਾ ਲਿਖਿਆ ਕੇਤਾ ਹੋਇ ॥

laykhā likhi-ā kaytā ho-i.

Just imagine what a huge scroll it would take!

ਕੇਤਾ ਤਾਣੁ ਸੁਆਲਿਹੁ ਰੂਪੁ ॥

kaytā tāṇ su-ālih(u) rūp.

What power! What fascinating beauty!

ਕੇਤੀ ਦਾਤਿ ਜਾਣੈ ਕੌਣੁ ਕੂਤੁ ॥

kaytī dāt jāṇai kauṇ kūt.

And what gifts! Who can know their extent?

ਕੀਤਾ ਪਸਾਉ ਏਕੋ ਕਵਾਉ ॥

kītā pasā-u ayko kavā-u.

You created the vast expanse of the Universe with One Word!

ਤਿਸ ਤੇ ਹੋਏ ਲਖ ਦਰੀਆਉ ॥

tis tay ho-ay lakh darī-ā-u.

Hundreds of thousands of rivers began to flow.

ਕੁਦਰਤਿ ਕਵਣ ਕਹਾ ਵੀਚਾਰੁ ॥

kudarat kavaṉ kahā vīchār.

How can Your Creative Potency be described?

ਵਾਰਿਆ ਨ ਜਾਵਾ ਏਕ ਵਾਰ ॥

vāri-ā na jāvā ayk vār.

I cannot even once be a sacrifice to You.

ਜੋ ਤੁਧੁ ਭਾਵੈ ਸਾਈ ਭਲੀ ਕਾਰ ॥

jo tudh bhāvai sā-ī bhalī kār.

Whatever pleases You is the only good done,

ਤੂ ਸਦਾ ਸਲਾਮਤਿ ਨਿਰੰਕਾਰ ॥੧੬॥

tū sadā salāmat nirankār. || 16||

You, Eternal and Formless One! || 16||

ਅਸੰਖ ਜਪ ਅਸੰਖ ਭਾਉ ॥

asankh jap asankh bhā-u.

Countless meditations, countless loves.

ਅਸੰਖ ਪੂਜਾ ਅਸੰਖ ਤਪ ਤਾਉ ॥

asankh pūjā asankh tap tā-u.

Countless worship services, countless austere disciplines.

ਅਸੰਖ ਗਰੰਥ ਮੁਖਿ ਵੇਦ ਪਾਠ ॥

asankh garanth mukh vayd pāṯh.

Countless scriptures, and ritual recitations of the Vedas.

ਅਸੰਖ ਜੋਗ ਮਨਿ ਰਹਹਿ ਉਦਾਸ ॥

asankh jog man rahah(i) udās.

Countless Yogīs, whose minds remain detached from the world.

ਅਸੰਖ ਭਗਤ ਗੁਣ ਗਿਆਨ ਵੀਚਾਰ ॥

asankh bhagat guṉ gi-ān vīchār.

Countless devotees contemplate the Wisdom and Virtues of the Lord.

ਅਸੰਖ ਸਤੀ ਅਸੰਖ ਦਾਤਾਰ ॥

asankh satī asankh dātār.

Countless the holy, countless the givers.

ਅਸੰਖ ਸੂਰ ਮੁਹ ਭਖ ਸਾਰ ॥

asankh sūr muh bhakh sār.

Countless heroic spiritual warriors, who bear the brunt of the attack in battle (who with their mouths eat steel).

ਅਸੰਖ ਮੋਨਿ ਲਿਵ ਲਾਇ ਤਾਰ ॥

asankh mon liv lā-i tār.

Countless silent sages, vibrating the String of His Love.

ਕੁਦਰਤਿ ਕਵਣ ਕਹਾ ਵੀਚਾਰੁ ॥

kudarat kavaṉ kahā vīchār.

How can Your Creative Potency be described?

ਵਾਰਿਆ ਨ ਜਾਵਾ ਏਕ ਵਾਰ ॥

vāri-ā na jāvā ayk vār.

I cannot even once be a sacrifice to You.

ਜੋ ਤੁਧੁ ਭਾਵੈ ਸਾਈ ਭਲੀ ਕਾਰ ॥

jo tudh bhāvai sā-ī bhalī kār.

Whatever pleases You is the only good done,

ਤੂ ਸਦਾ ਸਲਾਮਤਿ ਨਿਰੰਕਾਰ ॥੧੭॥

tū sadā salāmat nirankār. || 17||

You, Eternal and Formless One. || 17||

ਅਸੰਖ ਮੂਰਖ ਅੰਧ ਘੋਰ ॥

asankh mūrakh andh ghor.

Countless fools, blinded by ignorance.

ਅਸੰਖ ਚੋਰ ਹਰਾਮਖੋਰ ॥

asankh chor harāmakhor.

Countless thieves and embezzlers.

ਅਸੰਖ ਅਮਰ ਕਰਿ ਜਾਹਿ ਜੋਰ ॥

asankh amar kar jāh(i) jor.

Countless impose their will by force.

ਅਸੰਖ ਗਲਵਢ ਹਤਿਆ ਕਮਾਹਿ ॥

asankh galavadh hati-ā kamāh(i).

Countless cut-throats and ruthless killers.

ਅਸੰਖ ਪਾਪੀ ਪਾਪੁ ਕਰਿ ਜਾਹਿ ॥

asankh pāpī pāp kar jāh(i).

Countless sinners who keep on sinning.

ਅਸੰਖ ਕੂੜਿਆਰ ਕੂੜੇ ਫਿਰਾਹਿ ॥

asankh kūṛi-ār kūṛay phirāh(i).

Countless liars, wandering lost in their lies.

ਅਸੰਖ ਮਲੇਛ ਮਲੁ ਭਖਿ ਖਾਹਿ ॥

asankh malaychh mal bhakh khāh(i).

Countless wretches, eating filth as their ration.

ਅਸੰਖ ਨਿੰਦਕ ਸਿਰਿ ਕਰਹਿ ਭਾਰੁ ॥

asankh nindak sir karah(i) bhār.

Countless slanderers, carrying the weight of their stupid mistakes on their heads.

ਨਾਨਕੁ ਨੀਚੁ ਕਹੈ ਵੀਚਾਰੁ ॥

nānak nīch kahai vīchār.

Nānak describes the state of the lowly.

ਵਾਰਿਆ ਨ ਜਾਵਾ ਏਕ ਵਾਰ ॥

vāri-ā na jāvā ayk vār.

I cannot even once be a sacrifice to You.

ਜੋ ਤੁਧੁ ਭਾਵੈ ਸਾਈ ਭਲੀ ਕਾਰ ॥

jo tudh bhāvai sā-ī bhalī kār.

Whatever pleases You is the only good done,

ਤੂ ਸਦਾ ਸਲਾਮਤਿ ਨਿਰੰਕਾਰ ॥੧੮॥

tū sadā salāmat nirankār. || 18||

You, Eternal and Formless One. || 18||

ਅਸੰਖ ਨਾਵ ਅਸੰਖ ਥਾਵ ॥

asankh nāv asankh thāv.

Countless names, countless places.

ਅਗੰਮ ਅਗੰਮ ਅਸੰਖ ਲੋਅ ॥

agam agam asankh lo-a.

Inaccessible, unapproachable, countless celestial realms.

ਅਸੰਖ ਕਹਹਿ ਸਿਰਿ ਭਾਰੁ ਹੋਇ ॥

asankh kahah(i) sir bhār ho-i.

Even to call them countless is to carry the weight on your head.

ਅਖਰੀ ਨਾਮੁ ਅਖਰੀ ਸਾਲਾਹ ॥

akharī nām akharī sālāh.

From the Word, comes the Nām; from the Word, comes Your Praise.

ਅਖਰੀ ਗਿਆਨੁ ਗੀਤ ਗੁਣ ਗਾਹ ॥

akharī gi-ān gīt guṉ gāh.

From the Word, comes spiritual wisdom, singing the Songs of Your Glory.

ਅਖਰੀ ਲਿਖਣੁ ਬੋਲਣੁ ਬਾਣਿ ॥

akharī likhaṉ bolaṉ bāṉ.

From the Word, come the written and spoken words and hymns.

ਅਖਰਾ ਸਿਰਿ ਸੰਜੋਗੁ ਵਖਾਣਿ ॥

akharā sir sanjog vakhāṉ.

From the Word, comes destiny, written on one's forehead.

ਜਿਨਿ ਏਹਿ ਲਿਖੇ ਤਿਸੁ ਸਿਰਿ ਨਾਹਿ ॥

jin ayh(i) likhay tis sir nāh(i).

But the One who wrote these Words of Destiny—
no words are written on His Forehead.

ਜਿਵ ਫੁਰਮਾਏ ਤਿਵ ਤਿਵ ਪਾਹਿ ॥

jiv phuramā-ay tiv tiv pāh(i).

As He ordains, so do we receive.

ਜੇਤਾ ਕੀਤਾ ਤੇਤਾ ਨਾਉ ॥

jaytā kītā taytā nā-u.

The created universe is the manifestation of Your Name.

ਵਿਣੁ ਨਾਵੈ ਨਾਹੀ ਕੋ ਥਾਉ ॥

viṇ nāvai nāhī ko thā-u.

Without Your Name, there is no place at all.

ਕੁਦਰਤਿ ਕਵਣ ਕਹਾ ਵੀਚਾਰੁ ॥

kudarat kavaṇ kahā vīchār.

How can I describe Your Creative Power?

ਵਾਰਿਆ ਨ ਜਾਵਾ ਏਕ ਵਾਰ ॥

vāri-ā na jāvā ayk vār.

I cannot even once be a sacrifice to You.

ਜੋ ਤੁਧੁ ਭਾਵੈ ਸਾਈ ਭਲੀ ਕਾਰ ॥

jo tudh bhāvai sā-ī bhalī kār.

Whatever pleases You is the only good done,

ਤੂ ਸਦਾ ਸਲਾਮਤਿ ਨਿਰੰਕਾਰ ॥੧੯॥

tū sadā salāmat nirankār. || 19||

You, Eternal and Formless One. || 19||

ਭਰੀਐ ਹਥੁ ਪੈਰੁ ਤਨੁ ਦੇਹ ॥

bharī-ai hath pair tan dayh.

When the hands and the feet and the body are dirty,

ਪਾਣੀ ਧੋਤੈ ਉਤਰਸੁ ਖੇਹ ॥

pāṇī dhotai utaras khayh.

water can wash away the dirt.

ਮੂਤ ਪਲੀਤੀ ਕਪੜੁ ਹੋਇ ॥

mūt palītī kapaṛ ho-i.

When the clothes are soiled and stained by urine,

ਦੇ ਸਾਬੂਨੁ ਲਈਐ ਓਹੁ ਧੋਇ ॥

day sābūn la-ī-ai oh(u) dho-i.

soap can wash them clean.

ਭਰੀਐ ਮਤਿ ਪਾਪਾ ਕੈ ਸੰਗਿ ॥

bharī-ai mat pāpā kai sang.

But when the intellect is stained and polluted by sin,

ਓਹੁ ਧੋਪੈ ਨਾਵੈ ਕੈ ਰੰਗਿ ॥

oh(u) dhopai nāvai kai rang.

it can only be cleansed by the Love of the Name.

ਪੁੰਨੀ ਪਾਪੀ ਆਖਣੁ ਨਾਹਿ ॥

punī pāpī ākhan nāh(i).

Virtue and vice do not come by mere words;

ਕਰਿ ਕਰਿ ਕਰਣਾ ਲਿਖਿ ਲੈ ਜਾਹੁ ॥

kar kar karanā likh lai jāh(u).

actions repeated, over and over again, are engraved on the soul.

ਆਪੇ ਬੀਜਿ ਆਪੇ ਹੀ ਖਾਹੁ ॥

āpay bīj āpay hī khāh(u).

You shall harvest what you plant.

ਨਾਨਕ ਹੁਕਮੀ ਆਵਹੁ ਜਾਹੁ ॥੨੦॥

nānak hukamī āvah(u) jāh(u). ‖ 20‖

O Nānak, by the Hukam of God's Command,
we come and go in reincarnation. ‖20‖

ਤੀਰਥੁ ਤਪੁ ਦਇਆ ਦਤੁ ਦਾਨੁ ॥

tīrath tap da-i-ā dat dān.

Pilgrimages, austere discipline, compassion, and charity—

ਜੇ ਕੋ ਪਾਵੈ ਤਿਲ ਕਾ ਮਾਨੁ ॥

jay ko pāvai til kā mān.

these, by themselves, bring only an iota of merit.

ਸੁਣਿਆ ਮੰਨਿਆ ਮਨਿ ਕੀਤਾ ਭਾਉ ॥

suni-ā mani-ā man kītā bhā-u.

Listening and believing with love and humility in your mind,

ਅੰਤਰਗਤਿ ਤੀਰਥਿ ਮਲਿ ਨਾਉ ॥

antaragat tīrath mal nā-u.

cleanse yourself with the Name, at the sacred shrine deep within.

ਸਭਿ ਗੁਣ ਤੇਰੇ ਮੈ ਨਾਹੀ ਕੋਇ ॥

sabh gun tayray mai nāhī ko-i.

All virtues are Yours, Lord, I have none at all.

ਵਿਣੁ ਗੁਣ ਕੀਤੇ ਭਗਤਿ ਨ ਹੋਇ ॥

vin gun kītay bhagat na ho-i.

Without virtue, there is no devotional worship.

ਸੁਅਸਤਿ ਆਥਿ ਬਾਣੀ ਬਰਮਾਉ ॥

su-asat āth banī baramā-u.

I bow to the Lord of the World, to His Word, to Brahma the Creator.

ਸਤਿ ਸੁਹਾਣੁ ਸਦਾ ਮਨਿ ਚਾਉ ॥

sat suhān sadā man chā-u.

He is Beautiful, True, and Eternally Joyful.

ਕਵਣੁ ਸੁ ਵੇਲਾ ਵਖਤੁ ਕਵਣੁ ਕਵਣ ਥਿਤਿ ਕਵਣੁ ਵਾਰੁ ॥

kavaṉ su vaylā vakhat kavaṉ
kavaṉ thit kavaṉ vār.

What was that time, and what was that moment?
What was that day, and what was that date?

ਕਵਣਿ ਸਿ ਰੁਤੀ ਮਾਹੁ ਕਵਣੁ ਜਿਤੁ ਹੋਆ ਆਕਾਰੁ ॥

kavaṉ si rutī māh(u) kavaṉ jit ho-ā ākār.

What was that season, and what was that month, when the Universe was
created?

ਵੇਲ ਨ ਪਾਈਆ ਪੰਡਤੀ ਜਿ ਹੋਵੈ ਲੇਖੁ ਪੁਰਾਣੁ ॥

vayl na pā-ī-ā paṇḍatī ji hovai laykh purāṉ.

The Pandits, the religious scholars, cannot find that time,
even if it is written in the Purānas.

ਵਖਤੁ ਨ ਪਾਇਓ ਕਾਦੀਆ ਜਿ ਲਿਖਨਿ ਲੇਖੁ ਕੁਰਾਣੁ ॥

vakhat na pā-i-o kādī-ā ji likhan laykh kurāṉ.

That time is not known to the Qazis, who study the Koran.

ਥਿਤਿ ਵਾਰੁ ਨਾ ਜੋਗੀ ਜਾਣੈ ਰੁਤਿ ਮਾਹੁ ਨਾ ਕੋਈ ॥

thit vār nā jogī jāṉai rut māh(u) nā ko-ī.

The day and the date are not known to the Yogīs, nor is the month or the season.

ਜਾ ਕਰਤਾ ਸਿਰਠੀ ਕਉ ਸਾਜੇ ਆਪੇ ਜਾਣੈ ਸੋਈ ॥

jā karatā siraṭhī ka-u sājay āpay jāṉai so-ī.

The Creator who created this creation—only He Himself knows.

ਕਿਵ ਕਰਿ ਆਖਾ ਕਿਵ ਸਾਲਾਹੀ ਕਿਉ ਵਰਨੀ ਕਿਵ ਜਾਣਾ ॥

kiv kar ākhā kiv sālāhī ki-u varanī kiv jāṉā.

How can we speak of Him? How can we praise Him?
How can we describe Him? How can we know Him?

ਨਾਨਕ ਆਖਣਿ ਸਭੁ ਕੋ ਆਖੈ ਇਕ ਦੂ ਇਕੁ ਸਿਆਣਾ ॥

nānak ākhaṇ sabh ko ākhai ik dū ik si-āṇā.

O Nānak, everyone speaks of Him, each one wiser than the rest.

ਵਡਾ ਸਾਹਿਬੁ ਵਡੀ ਨਾਈ ਕੀਤਾ ਜਾ ਕਾ ਹੋਵੈ ॥

vaḍā sāhib vaḍī nā-ī kītā jā kā hovai.

Great is the Master, Great is His Name.
Whatever happens is according to His Will.

ਨਾਨਕ ਜੇ ਕੋ ਆਪੌ ਜਾਣੈ ਅਗੈ ਗਇਆ ਨ ਸੋਹੈ ॥੨੧॥

nānak jay ko āpau jāṇai agai ga-i-ā na sohai. ॥21॥

O Nānak, one who claims to know everything shall not be decorated
in the world hereafter. ॥21॥

ਪਾਤਾਲਾ ਪਾਤਾਲ ਲਖ ਆਗਾਸਾ ਆਗਾਸ ॥

pātālā pātāl lakh āgāsā āgās.

There are netherworlds beneath netherworlds,
and hundreds of thousands of heavenly worlds above.

ਓੜਕ ਓੜਕ ਭਾਲਿ ਥਕੇ ਵੇਦ ਕਹਨਿ ਇਕ ਵਾਤ ॥

oṛak oṛak bhāl thakay vayd kahan ik vāt.

The Vedas say that you can search and search for them all, until you grow weary.

ਸਹਸ ਅਠਾਰਹ ਕਹਨਿ ਕਤੇਬਾ ਅਸੁਲੂ ਇਕੁ ਧਾਤੁ ॥

sahas aṭhārah kahan kataybā asulū ik dhāt.

The scriptures say that there are 18,000 worlds, but in reality,
there is only One Universe.

ਲੇਖਾ ਹੋਇ ਤ ਲਿਖੀਐ ਲੇਖੈ ਹੋਇ ਵਿਣਾਸੁ ॥

laykhā ho-i ta likhī-ai laykhai ho-i viṇās.

If you try to write an account of this, you will surely finish yourself
before you finish writing it.

185

ਨਾਨਕ ਵਡਾ ਆਖੀਐ ਆਪੇ ਜਾਣੈ ਆਪੁ ॥੨੨॥

nānak vaḍā ākhī-ai āpay jāṇai āp. || 22||

O Nānak, call Him Great! He Himself knows Himself. || 22||

ਸਾਲਾਹੀ ਸਾਲਾਹਿ ਏਤੀ ਸੁਰਤਿ ਨ ਪਾਈਆ ॥

sālāhī sālāh(i) aytī surat na pā-ī-ā.

The praisers praise the Lord, but they do not obtain intuitive understanding—

ਨਦੀਆ ਅਤੈ ਵਾਹ ਪਵਹਿ ਸਮੁੰਦਿ ਨ ਜਾਣੀਅਹਿ ॥

nadī-ā atai vāh pavah(i) samund na jāṇī-ah(i).

the streams and rivers flowing into the ocean do not know its vastness.

ਸਮੁੰਦ ਸਾਹ ਸੁਲਤਾਨ ਗਿਰਹਾ ਸੇਤੀ ਮਾਲੁ ਧਨੁ ॥

samund sāh sulatān girahā saytī māl dhan.

Even kings and emperors, with mountains of property and oceans of wealth—

ਕੀੜੀ ਤੁਲਿ ਨ ਹੋਵਨੀ ਜੇ ਤਿਸੁ ਮਨਹੁ ਨ ਵੀਸਰਹਿ ॥੨੩॥

kīṛī tul na hovanī jay tis manah(u) na vīsarah(i). || 23||

these are not even equal to an ant, who does not forget God. || 23||

ਅੰਤੁ ਨ ਸਿਫਤੀ ਕਹਣਿ ਨ ਅੰਤੁ ॥

ant na siphatī kahaṇ na ant.

Endless are His Praises, endless are those who speak them.

ਅੰਤੁ ਨ ਕਰਣੈ ਦੇਣਿ ਨ ਅੰਤੁ ॥

ant na karaṇai dayṇ na ant.

Endless are His Actions, endless are His Gifts.

ਅੰਤੁ ਨ ਵੇਖਣਿ ਸੁਣਣਿ ਨ ਅੰਤੁ ॥

ant na vaykhaṇ suṇaṇ na ant.

Endless is His Vision, endless is His Hearing.

ਅੰਤੁ ਨ ਜਾਪੈ ਕਿਆ ਮਨਿ ਮੰਤੁ ॥

ant na jāpai ki-ā man mant.

His limits cannot be perceived. What is the Mystery of His Mind?

ਅੰਤੁ ਨ ਜਾਪੈ ਕੀਤਾ ਆਕਾਰੁ ॥

ant na jāpai kītā ākār.

The limits of the created universe cannot be perceived.

ਅੰਤੁ ਨ ਜਾਪੈ ਪਾਰਾਵਾਰੁ ॥

ant na jāpai pārāvār.

Its limits here and beyond cannot be perceived.

ਅੰਤ ਕਾਰਣਿ ਕੇਤੇ ਬਿਲਲਾਹਿ ॥

ant kāraṉ kaytay bilalāh(i).

Many struggle to know His limits,

ਤਾ ਕੇ ਅੰਤ ਨ ਪਾਏ ਜਾਹਿ ॥

tā kay ant na pā-ay jāh(i).

but His limits cannot be found.

ਏਹੁ ਅੰਤੁ ਨ ਜਾਣੈ ਕੋਇ ॥

ayh(u) ant na jāṉai ko-i.

No one can know these limits.

ਬਹੁਤਾ ਕਹੀਐ ਬਹੁਤਾ ਹੋਇ ॥

bahutā kahī-ai bahutā ho-i.

The more you say about them, the more there still remains to be said.

ਵਡਾ ਸਾਹਿਬੁ ਊਚਾ ਥਾਉ ॥

vaḍā sāhib ūchā thā-u.

Great is the Master, High is His Heavenly Home.

ਉਚੇ ਉਪਰਿ ਉਚਾ ਨਾਉ ॥

ūchay upar ūchā nā-u.

Highest of the High, above all is His Name.

ਏਵਡੁ ਉਚਾ ਹੋਵੈ ਕੋਇ ॥

ayvad ūchā hovai ko-i.

Only one as Great and as High as God

ਤਿਸੁ ਉਚੇ ਕਉ ਜਾਣੈ ਸੋਇ ॥

tis ūchay ka-u jāṇai so-i.

can know His Lofty and Exalted State.

ਜੇਵਡੁ ਆਪਿ ਜਾਣੈ ਆਪਿ ਆਪਿ ॥

jayvad āp jāṇai āp āp.

Only He Himself is that Great. He Himself knows Himself.

ਨਾਨਕ ਨਦਰੀ ਕਰਮੀ ਦਾਤਿ ॥੨੪॥

nānak nadarī karamī dāt. || 24||

O Nānak, by His Glance of Grace, He bestows His Blessings. ||24||

ਬਹੁਤਾ ਕਰਮੁ ਲਿਖਿਆ ਨਾ ਜਾਇ ॥

bahutā karam likhi-ā nā jā-i.

His Blessings are so abundant that there can be no written account of them.

ਵਡਾ ਦਾਤਾ ਤਿਲੁ ਨ ਤਮਾਇ ॥

vadā dātā til na tamā-i.

The Great Giver does not hold back anything.

ਕੇਤੇ ਮੰਗਹਿ ਜੋਧ ਅਪਾਰ ॥

kaytay mangah(i) jodh apār.

There are so many great, heroic warriors begging at the Door of the Infinite Lord.

ਕੇਤਿਆ ਗਣਤ ਨਹੀ ਵੀਚਾਰੁ ॥

kayti-ā ganat nahī vīchār.

So many contemplate and dwell upon Him that they cannot be counted.

ਕੇਤੇ ਖਪਿ ਤੁਟਹਿ ਵੇਕਾਰ ॥

kaytay khap tutah(i) vaykār.

So many waste away to death engaged in corruption.

ਕੇਤੇ ਲੈ ਲੈ ਮੁਕਰੁ ਪਾਹਿ ॥

kaytay lai lai mukar pāh(i).

So many take and take again, and then deny receiving.

ਕੇਤੇ ਮੂਰਖ ਖਾਹੀ ਖਾਹਿ ॥

kaytay mūrakh khāhī khāh(i).

So many foolish consumers keep on consuming.

ਕੇਤਿਆ ਦੂਖ ਭੂਖ ਸਦ ਮਾਰ ॥

kayti-ā dūkh bhūkh sad mār.

So many endure distress, deprivation, and constant abuse.

ਏਹਿ ਭਿ ਦਾਤਿ ਤੇਰੀ ਦਾਤਾਰ ॥

ayh(i) bhi dāt tayrī dātār.

Even these are Your Gifts, O Great Giver!

ਬੰਦਿ ਖਲਾਸੀ ਭਾਣੈ ਹੋਇ ॥

band khalāsī bhānai ho-i.

Liberation from bondage comes only by Your Will.

ਹੋਰੁ ਆਖਿ ਨ ਸਕੈ ਕੋਇ ॥

hor ākh na sakai ko-i.

No one else has any say in this.

189

ਜੇ ਕੋ ਖਾਇਕੁ ਆਖਣਿ ਪਾਇ ॥

jay ko khā-ik ākhaṇ pā-i.

If some fool should presume to say that he does,

ਓਹੁ ਜਾਣੈ ਜੇਤੀਆ ਮੁਹਿ ਖਾਇ ॥

oh(u) jāṇai jaytī-ā muh(i) khā-i.

he shall learn and feel the effects of his folly.

ਆਪੇ ਜਾਣੈ ਆਪੇ ਦੇਇ ॥

āpay jāṇai āpay day-i.

He Himself knows, He Himself gives.

ਆਖਹਿ ਸਿ ਭਿ ਕੇਈ ਕੇਇ ॥

ākhah(i) si bhi kay-ī kay-i.

Few, very few are those who acknowledge this.

ਜਿਸ ਨੋ ਬਖਸੇ ਸਿਫਤਿ ਸਾਲਾਹ ॥

jis no bakhasay siphat sālāh.

One who is blessed to sing the Praises of the Lord,

ਨਾਨਕ ਪਾਤਿਸਾਹੀ ਪਾਤਿਸਾਹੁ ॥੨੫॥

nānak pātisāhī pātisāh(u). ‖25‖

O Nānak, is the king of kings. ‖25‖

ਅਮੁਲ ਗੁਣ ਅਮੁਲ ਵਾਪਾਰ ॥

amul guṇ amul vāpār.

Priceless are His Virtues, Priceless are His Dealings.

ਅਮੁਲ ਵਾਪਾਰੀਏ ਅਮੁਲ ਭੰਡਾਰ ॥

amul vāpārī-ay amul bhandār.

Priceless are His Dealers, Priceless are His Treasures.

ਅਮੁਲ ਆਵਹਿ ਅਮੁਲ ਲੈ ਜਾਹਿ ॥

amul āvah(i) amul lai jāh(i).

Priceless are those who come to Him, Priceless are those who buy from Him.

ਅਮੁਲ ਭਾਇ ਅਮੁਲਾ ਸਮਾਹਿ ॥

amul bhā-i amulā samāh(i).

Priceless is Love for Him, Priceless is absorption into Him.

ਅਮੁਲੁ ਧਰਮੁ ਅਮੁਲੁ ਦੀਬਾਣੁ ॥

amul dharam amul dībāṇ.

Priceless is the Divine Law of Dharma, Priceless is the Divine Court of Justice.

ਅਮੁਲੁ ਤੁਲੁ ਅਮੁਲੁ ਪਰਵਾਣੁ ॥

amul tul amul paravāṇ.

Priceless are the scales, priceless are the weights.

ਅਮੁਲੁ ਬਖਸੀਸ ਅਮੁਲੁ ਨੀਸਾਣੁ ॥

amul bakhasīs amul nīsāṇ.

Priceless are His Blessings, Priceless is His Banner and Insignia.

ਅਮੁਲੁ ਕਰਮੁ ਅਮੁਲੁ ਫੁਰਮਾਣੁ ॥

amul karam amul phuramāṇ.

Priceless is His Mercy, Priceless is His Royal Command.

ਅਮੁਲੋ ਅਮੁਲੁ ਆਖਿਆ ਨ ਜਾਇ ॥

amulo amul ākhi-ā na jā-i.

Priceless, O Priceless beyond expression!

ਆਖਿ ਆਖਿ ਰਹੇ ਲਿਵ ਲਾਇ ॥

ākh ākh rahay liv lā-i.

Speak of Him continually, and remain absorbed in His Love.

ਆਖਹਿ ਵੇਦ ਪਾਠ ਪੁਰਾਣ ॥

ākhah(i) vayd pāṯẖ purān̲.

The Vedas and the Purānas speak.

ਆਖਹਿ ਪੜੇ ਕਰਹਿ ਵਖਿਆਣ ॥

ākhah(i) paṛay karah(i) vakhi-ān̲.

The scholars speak and lecture.

ਆਖਹਿ ਬਰਮੇ ਆਖਹਿ ਇੰਦ ॥

ākhah(i) baramay ākhah(i) ind.

Brahma speaks, Indra speaks.

ਆਖਹਿ ਗੋਪੀ ਤੈ ਗੋਵਿੰਦ ॥

ākhah(i) gopī tai govind.

The Gopis and Krishna speak.

ਆਖਹਿ ਈਸਰ ਆਖਹਿ ਸਿਧ ॥

ākhah(i) īsar ākhah(i) sidh.

Shiva speaks, the Siddhas speak.

ਆਖਹਿ ਕੇਤੇ ਕੀਤੇ ਬੁਧ ॥

ākhah(i) kaytay kītay budh.

The many created Buddhas speak.

ਆਖਹਿ ਦਾਨਵ ਆਖਹਿ ਦੇਵ ॥

ākhah(i) dānav ākhah(i) dayv.

The demons speak, the demi-gods speak.

ਆਖਹਿ ਸੁਰਿ ਨਰ ਮੁਨਿ ਜਨ ਸੇਵ ॥

ākhah(i) sur nar mun jan sayv.

*The spiritual warriors, the heavenly beings, the silent sages,
the humble and serviceful speak.*

ਕੇਤੇ ਆਖਹਿ ਆਖਣਿ ਪਾਹਿ ॥

kaytay ākhah(i) ākhan pāhi.

Many speak and try to describe Him.

ਕੇਤੇ ਕਹਿ ਕਹਿ ਉਠਿ ਉਠਿ ਜਾਹਿ ॥

kaytay kah(i) kah(i) uth uth jāh(i).

Many have spoken of Him over and over again,
and have then arisen and departed.

ਏਤੇ ਕੀਤੇ ਹੋਰਿ ਕਰੇਹਿ ॥

aytay kītay hor(i) karayh(i).

If He were to create as many again as there already are,

ਤਾ ਆਖਿ ਨ ਸਕਹਿ ਕੇਈ ਕੇਇ ॥

tā ākh na sakah(i) kay-ī kay-i.

even then, they could not describe Him.

ਜੇਵਡੁ ਭਾਵੈ ਤੇਵਡੁ ਹੋਇ ॥

jayvad bhāvai tayvad ho-i.

He is as Great as He wishes to be.

ਨਾਨਕ ਜਾਣੈ ਸਾਚਾ ਸੋਇ ॥

nānak jānai sāchā so-i.

O Nānak, the True Lord knows.

ਜੇ ਕੋ ਆਖੈ ਬੋਲੁਵਿਗਾੜੁ ॥

jay ko ākhai boluvigāṛ.

If anyone presumes to describe God,

ਤਾ ਲਿਖੀਐ ਸਿਰਿ ਗਾਵਾਰਾ ਗਾਵਾਰੁ ॥੨੬॥

tā likī-ai sir gāvārā gāvār. || 26||

he shall be known as the greatest fool of fools! ||26||

ਸੋ ਦਰੁ ਕੇਹਾ ਸੋ ਘਰੁ ਕੇਹਾ ਜਿਤੁ ਬਹਿ ਸਰਬ ਸਮਾਲੇ ॥

so dar kayhā so ghar kayhā jit bah(i) sarab samālay.

Where is that Gate, and where is that Dwelling,
in which You sit and take care of all?

ਵਾਜੇ ਨਾਦ ਅਨੇਕ ਅਸੰਖਾ ਕੇਤੇ ਵਾਵਣਹਾਰੇ ॥

vājay nād anayk asankhā kaytay vāvaṇahāray.

The Sound Current of the Naad vibrates there,
and countless musicians play on all sorts of instruments there.

ਕੇਤੇ ਰਾਗ ਪਰੀ ਸਿਉ ਕਹੀਅਨਿ ਕੇਤੇ ਗਾਵਣਹਾਰੇ ॥

kaytay rāg parī si-u kahī-an kaytay gāvaṇahāray.

So many Ragas, so many musicians singing there.

ਗਾਵਹਿ ਤੁਹਨੋ ਪਉਣੁ ਪਾਣੀ ਬੈਸੰਤਰੁ ਗਾਵੈ ਰਾਜਾ ਧਰਮੁ ਦੁਆਰੇ ॥

gāvah(i) tuhano pa-uṇ pāṇī baisantar
gāvai rājā dharam du-āray.

The prānic wind, water and fire sing;
the Righteous Judge of Dharma sings at Your Door.

ਗਾਵਹਿ ਚਿਤੁ ਗੁਪਤੁ ਲਿਖਿ ਜਾਣਹਿ ਲਿਖਿ ਲਿਖਿ ਧਰਮੁ ਵੀਚਾਰੇ ॥

gāvah(i) chit gupat likh jāṇah(i)
likh likh dharam vīchāray.

Chitr and Gupat, the angels of the conscious and the subconscious who record
actions, and the Righteous Judge of Dharma who judges this record sing.

ਗਾਵਹਿ ਈਸਰੁ ਬਰਮਾ ਦੇਵੀ ਸੋਹਨਿ ਸਦਾ ਸਵਾਰੇ ॥

gāvah(i) īsar baramā dayvī sohan sadā savāray.

Shiva, Brahma, and the Goddess of Beauty, ever adorned, sing.

ਗਾਵਹਿ ਇੰਦ ਇਦਾਸਣਿ ਬੈਠੇ ਦੇਵਤਿਆ ਦਰਿ ਨਾਲੇ ॥

gāvah(i) ind idāsaṇ baiṭhay dayvati-ā dar nālay.

Indra, seated upon the Throne, sings with the deities at Your Door.

194

ਗਾਵਹਿ ਸਿਧ ਸਮਾਧੀ ਅੰਦਰਿ ਗਾਵਨਿ ਸਾਧ ਵਿਚਾਰੇ ॥

gāvah(i) sidh samādhī andar gāvan sādh vichāray.

The Siddhas in Samādhi sing; the Sādhus sing in contemplation.

ਗਾਵਨਿ ਜਤੀ ਸਤੀ ਸੰਤੋਖੀ ਗਾਵਹਿ ਵੀਰ ਕਰਾਰੇ ॥

gāvan jatī satī santokhī gāvah(i) vīr karāray.

The celibates, the fanatics, the peacefully accepting, and the fearless warriors sing.

ਗਾਵਨਿ ਪੰਡਿਤ ਪੜਨਿ ਰਖੀਸਰ ਜੁਗੁ ਜੁਗੁ ਵੇਦਾ ਨਾਲੇ ॥

gāvan pandit paran rakhīsar jug jug vaydā nālay.

*The Pandits, the religious scholars who recite the Vedas,
with the supreme sages of all the ages, sing.*

ਗਾਵਹਿ ਮੋਹਣੀਆ ਮਨੁ ਮੋਹਨਿ ਸੁਰਗਾ ਮਛ ਪਇਆਲੇ ॥

gāvah(i) mohanī-ā man mohan suragā machh pa-i-ālay.

*The Mohīnīs, the enchanting heavenly beauties who entice hearts in this world,
in paradise, and in the underworld of the subconscious, sing.*

ਗਾਵਨਿ ਰਤਨ ਉਪਾਏ ਤੇਰੇ ਅਠਸਠਿ ਤੀਰਥ ਨਾਲੇ ॥

gāvan ratan upā-ay tayray athasath tīrath nālay.

*The celestial jewels created by You,
and the sixty-eight holy places of pilgrimage sing.*

ਗਾਵਹਿ ਜੋਧ ਮਹਾਬਲ ਸੂਰਾ ਗਾਵਹਿ ਖਾਣੀ ਚਾਰੇ ॥

gāvah(i) jodh mahābal sūrā gāvah(i) khānī chāray.

*The brave and mighty warriors sing;
the spiritual heroes and the four sources of creation sing.*

ਗਾਵਹਿ ਖੰਡ ਮੰਡਲ ਵਰਭੰਡਾ ਕਰਿ ਕਰਿ ਰਖੇ ਧਾਰੇ ॥

gāvah(i) khand mandal varabhandā kar kar rakhay dhāray.

*The planets, solar systems, and galaxies, created and arranged
by Your Hand, sing.*

ਸੇਈ ਤੁਧੁਨੋ ਗਾਵਹਿ ਜੋ ਤੁਧੁ ਭਾਵਨਿ ਰਤੇ ਤੇਰੇ ਭਗਤ ਰਸਾਲੇ ॥

say-ī tudhuno gāvah(i) jo tudh bhāvan
ratay tayray bhagat rasālay.

They alone sing, who are pleasing to Your Will.
Your devotees are imbued with the Nectar of Your Essence.

ਹੋਰਿ ਕੇਤੇ ਗਾਵਨਿ ਸੇ ਮੈ ਚਿਤਿ ਨ ਆਵਨਿ ਨਾਨਕੁ ਕਿਆ ਵੀਚਾਰੇ ॥

hor kaytay gāvan say mai chit na āvan
nānak ki-ā vīchāray.

So many others sing, they do not come to mind.
O Nānak, how can I consider them all?

ਸੋਈ ਸੋਈ ਸਦਾ ਸਚੁ ਸਾਹਿਬੁ ਸਾਚਾ ਸਾਚੀ ਨਾਈ ॥

so-ī so-ī sadā sach sāhib sāchā sāchī nā-ī.

That True Lord is True, Forever True, and True is His Name.

ਹੈ ਭੀ ਹੋਸੀ ਜਾਇ ਨ ਜਾਸੀ ਰਚਨਾ ਜਿਨਿ ਰਚਾਈ ॥

hai bhī hosī jā-i na jāsī rachanā jin rachā-ī.

He is, and shall always be. He shall not depart,
even when this Universe which He has created departs.

ਰੰਗੀ ਰੰਗੀ ਭਾਤੀ ਕਰਿ ਕਰਿ ਜਿਨਸੀ ਮਾਇਆ ਜਿਨਿ ਉਪਾਈ ॥

rangī rangī bhātī kar kar jinasī mā-i-ā jin upā-ī.

He created the world, with its various colors,
species of beings, and the variety of Maya.

ਕਰਿ ਕਰਿ ਵੇਖੈ ਕੀਤਾ ਆਪਣਾ ਜਿਵ ਤਿਸ ਦੀ ਵਡਿਆਈ ॥

kar kar vaykhai kītā āpaṇā jiv tis dī vaḍi-ā-ī.

Having created the creation, He watches over it Himself, by His Greatness.

ਜੋ ਤਿਸੁ ਭਾਵੈ ਸੋਈ ਕਰਸੀ ਹੁਕਮੁ ਨ ਕਰਣਾ ਜਾਈ ॥

jo tis bhāvai so-ī karasī hukam na karaṇā jā-ī.

He does whatever He pleases. No order can be issued to Him.

ਸੋ ਪਾਤਿਸਾਹੁ ਸਾਹਾ ਪਾਤਿਸਾਹਿਬੁ ਨਾਨਕ ਰਹਣੁ ਰਜਾਈ ॥੨੭॥

so pātisāh(u) sāhā pātisāhib nānak rahaṇ rajā-ī. ‖27‖

He is the King, the King of kings, the Supreme Lord and Master of kings.
Nānak remains subject to His Will. ‖27‖

ਮੁੰਦਾ ਸੰਤੋਖੁ ਸਰਮੁ ਪਤੁ ਝੋਲੀ ਧਿਆਨ ਕੀ ਕਰਹਿ ਬਿਭੂਤਿ ॥

munda santokh saram pat jholī
dhi-ān kī karah(i) bibhūt.

Make contentment your earrings, humility your begging bowl,
and meditation the ashes you apply to your body.

ਖਿੰਥਾ ਕਾਲੁ ਕੁਆਰੀ ਕਾਇਆ ਜੁਗਤਿ ਡੰਡਾ ਪਰਤੀਤਿ ॥

khinthā kāl ku-ārī kā-i-ā jugat ḍaṇḍā paratīt.

Let the remembrance of death be the patched coat you wear,
let the purity of virginity be your way in the world,
and let faith in the Lord be your walking stick.

ਆਈ ਪੰਥੀ ਸਗਲ ਜਮਾਤੀ ਮਨਿ ਜੀਤੈ ਜਗੁ ਜੀਤੁ ॥

ā-ī panthī sagal jamātī man jītai jag jīt.

See the brotherhood of all mankind as the highest order of Yogīs;
conquer your own mind, and conquer the world.

ਆਦੇਸੁ ਤਿਸੈ ਆਦੇਸੁ ॥

ādays tisai ādays.

I bow to Him, I humbly bow.

ਆਦਿ ਅਨੀਲੁ ਅਨਾਦਿ ਅਨਾਹਤਿ ਜੁਗੁ ਜੁਗੁ ਏਕੋ ਵੇਸੁ ॥੨੮॥

ād anīl anād anāhat jug jug ayko vays. ‖28‖

The Primal One, the Pure Light, without beginning, without end.
Throughout all the ages, He is One and the Same. ‖28‖

ਭੁਗਤਿ ਗਿਆਨੁ ਦਇਆ ਭੰਡਾਰਣਿ ਘਟਿ ਘਟਿ ਵਾਜਹਿ ਨਾਦ ॥

bhugat gi-ān da-i-ā bhandāran ghat ghat vājah(i) nād.

Let spiritual wisdom be your food, and compassion your attendant.
The Sound Current of the Naad vibrates in each and every heart.

ਆਪਿ ਨਾਥੁ ਨਾਥੀ ਸਭ ਜਾ ਕੀ ਰਿਧਿ ਸਿਧਿ ਅਵਰਾ ਸਾਦ ॥

āp nāth nāthī sabh jā kī ridh sidh avarā sād.

He Himself is the Supreme Master of all; wealth and miraculous spiritual
powers,
and all other external tastes and pleasures, are all like beads on a string.

ਸੰਜੋਗੁ ਵਿਜੋਗੁ ਦੁਇ ਕਾਰ ਚਲਾਵਹਿ ਲੇਖੇ ਆਵਹਿ ਭਾਗ ॥

sanjog vijog du-i kār chalāvah(i) laykhay āvah(i) bhāg.

Union with Him, and separation from Him, come by His Will.
We come to receive what is written in our destiny.

ਆਦੇਸੁ ਤਿਸੈ ਆਦੇਸੁ ॥

ādays tisai ādays.

I bow to Him, I humbly bow.

ਆਦਿ ਅਨੀਲੁ ਅਨਾਦਿ ਅਨਾਹਤਿ ਜੁਗੁ ਜੁਗੁ ਏਕੋ ਵੇਸੁ ॥੨੯॥

ād anīl anād anāhat jug jug ayko vays. || 29||

The Primal One, the Pure Light, without beginning, without end.
Throughout all the ages, He is One and the Same. ||29||

ਏਕਾ ਮਾਈ ਜੁਗਤਿ ਵਿਆਈ ਤਿਨਿ ਚੇਲੇ ਪਰਵਾਣੁ ॥

aykā mā-ī jugat vi-ā-ī tin chaylay paravān.

The One Divine Mother conceived and gave birth to the three deities.

ਇਕੁ ਸੰਸਾਰੀ ਇਕੁ ਭੰਡਾਰੀ ਇਕੁ ਲਾਏ ਦੀਬਾਣੁ ॥

ik sansārī ik bhandārī ik lā-ay dībān.

One, the Creator of the World; One, the Sustainer; and One, the Destroyer.

ਜਿਵ ਤਿਸੁ ਭਾਵੈ ਤਿਵੈ ਚਲਾਵੈ ਜਿਵ ਹੋਵੈ ਫੁਰਮਾਣੁ ॥

jiv tis bhāvai tivai chalāvai jiv hovai phuramāṇ.

God makes things happen according to the Pleasure of God's Will.
Such is God's Celestial Order.

ਓਹੁ ਵੇਖੈ ਓਨਾ ਨਦਰਿ ਨ ਆਵੈ ਬਹੁਤਾ ਏਹੁ ਵਿਡਾਣੁ ॥

oh(u) vaykhai onā nadar na āvai bahutā ayh(u) viḍāṇ.

God watches over all, but none see God. How wonderful this is!

ਆਦੇਸੁ ਤਿਸੈ ਆਦੇਸੁ ॥

ādays tisai ādays.

I bow to Him, I humbly bow.

ਆਦਿ ਅਨੀਲੁ ਅਨਾਦਿ ਅਨਾਹਤਿ ਜੁਗੁ ਜੁਗੁ ਏਕੋ ਵੇਸੁ ॥੩੦॥

ād anīl anād anāhat jug jug ayko vays. || 30||

The Primal One, the Pure Light, without beginning, without end.
Throughout all the ages, He is One and the Same. ||30||

ਆਸਣੁ ਲੋਇ ਲੋਇ ਭੰਡਾਰ ॥

āsan lo-i lo-i bhanḍār.

On world after world are His Seats of Authority and His Storehouses.

ਜੋ ਕਿਛੁ ਪਾਇਆ ਸੁ ਏਕਾ ਵਾਰ ॥

jo kichh pā-i-ā su aykā vār.

Whatever was put into them, was put there once and for all.

ਕਰਿ ਕਰਿ ਵੇਖੈ ਸਿਰਜਣਹਾਰੁ ॥

kar kar vaykhai sirajaṇahār.

Having created the creation, the Creator Lord watches over it.

ਨਾਨਕ ਸਚੇ ਕੀ ਸਾਚੀ ਕਾਰ ॥

nānak sachay kī sāchī kār.

O Nānak, True is the Creation of the True Lord.

ਆਦੇਸੁ ਤਿਸੈ ਆਦੇਸੁ ॥

ādays tisai ādays.

I bow to Him, I humbly bow.

ਆਦਿ ਅਨੀਲੁ ਅਨਾਦਿ ਅਨਾਹਤਿ ਜੁਗੁ ਜੁਗੁ ਏਕੋ ਵੇਸੁ ॥੩੧॥

ād anīl anād anāhat jug jug ayko vays. || 31||

The Primal One, the Pure Light, without beginning, without end.
Throughout all the ages, He is One and the Same. ||31||

ਇਕ ਦੂ ਜੀਭੌ ਲਖ ਹੋਹਿ ਲਖ ਹੋਵਹਿ ਲਖ ਵੀਸ ॥

ik dū jībhau lakh hoh(i) lakh hovah(i) lakh vīs.

If I had 100,000 tongues, and these were then multiplied twenty times more,
with each tongue,

ਲਖੁ ਲਖੁ ਗੇੜਾ ਆਖੀਅਹਿ ਏਕੁ ਨਾਮੁ ਜਗਦੀਸ ॥

lakh lakh gayṟā ākhī-ah(i) ayk nām jagadīs.

I would repeat, hundreds of thousands of times, the Name of the One,
the Lord of the Universe.

ਏਤੁ ਰਾਹਿ ਪਤਿ ਪਵੜੀਆ ਚੜੀਐ ਹੋਇ ਇਕੀਸ ॥

ayt rāh(i) pat pavaṟī-ā chaṟī-ai ho-i ikīs.

Along this path to our Husband Lord, we climb the steps of the ladder,
and come to merge with Him.

ਸੁਣਿ ਗਲਾ ਆਕਾਸ ਕੀ ਕੀਟਾ ਆਈ ਰੀਸ ॥

suṉ galā ākās kī kīṭā ā-ī rīs.

Hearing of the etheric realms, even worms long to come back home.

ਨਾਨਕ ਨਦਰੀ ਪਾਈਐ ਕੂੜੀ ਕੂੜੈ ਠੀਸ ॥੩੨॥

nānak nadarī pā-ī-ai kūṛī kūṛai ṭhīs. || 32||

O Nānak, by His Grace He is obtained. False are the boastings of the false. ||32||

ਆਖਣਿ ਜੋਰੁ ਚੁਪੈ ਨਹ ਜੋਰੁ ॥

ākhaṇ jor chupai nah jor.

No power to speak, no power to keep silent.

ਜੋਰੁ ਨ ਮੰਗਣਿ ਦੇਣਿ ਨ ਜੋਰੁ ॥

jor na mangaṇ dayṇ na jor.

No power to beg, no power to give.

ਜੋਰੁ ਨ ਜੀਵਣਿ ਮਰਣਿ ਨਹ ਜੋਰੁ ॥

jor na jīvaṇ maraṇ nah jor.

No power to live, no power to die.

ਜੋਰੁ ਨ ਰਾਜਿ ਮਾਲਿ ਮਨਿ ਸੋਰੁ ॥

jor na rāj māl man sor.

No power to rule, with wealth and occult mental powers.

ਜੋਰੁ ਨ ਸੁਰਤੀ ਗਿਆਨਿ ਵੀਚਾਰਿ ॥

jor na suratī gi-ān vīchār.

No power to gain intuitive understanding, spiritual wisdom, and meditation.

ਜੋਰੁ ਨ ਜੁਗਤੀ ਛੁਟੈ ਸੰਸਾਰੁ ॥

jor na jugatī chhuṭai sansār.

No power to find the way to escape from the world.

ਜਿਸੁ ਹਥਿ ਜੋਰੁ ਕਰਿ ਵੇਖੈ ਸੋਇ ॥

jis hath jor kar vaykhai so-i.

He alone has the Power in His Hands. He watches over all.

ਨਾਨਕ ਉਤਮੁ ਨੀਚੁ ਨ ਕੋਇ ॥੩੩॥

nānak utam nīch na ko-i. || 33||

O Nānak, no one is high or low. ||33||

ਰਾਤੀ ਰੁਤੀ ਥਿਤੀ ਵਾਰ ॥

rātī rutī thitī vār.

Nights, days, weeks, and seasons;

ਪਵਣ ਪਾਣੀ ਅਗਨੀ ਪਾਤਾਲ ॥

pavaṇ pāṇī aganī pātāl.

wind, water, fire, and the nether regions—

ਤਿਸੁ ਵਿਚਿ ਧਰਤੀ ਥਾਪਿ ਰਖੀ ਧਰਮ ਸਾਲ ॥

tis vich dharatī thāp rakhī dharam sāl.

in the midst of these, He established the earth as a home for Dharma.

ਤਿਸੁ ਵਿਚਿ ਜੀਅ ਜੁਗਤਿ ਕੇ ਰੰਗ ॥

tis vich jī-a jugat kay rang.

Upon it, He placed the various species of beings.

ਤਿਨ ਕੇ ਨਾਮ ਅਨੇਕ ਅਨੰਤ ॥

tin kay nām anayk anant.

Their names are uncounted and endless.

ਕਰਮੀ ਕਰਮੀ ਹੋਇ ਵੀਚਾਰੁ ॥

karamī karamī ho-i vīchār.

By their deeds and their actions, they shall be judged.

ਸਚਾ ਆਪਿ ਸਚਾ ਦਰਬਾਰੁ ॥

sachā āp sachā darabār.

God Himself is True, and True is His Court.

ਤਿਥੈ ਸੋਹਨਿ ਪੰਚ ਪਰਵਾਣੁ ॥

tithai sohan panch paravāṇ.

There, in perfect grace and ease, sit the self-elect, the self-realized Saints.

ਨਦਰੀ ਕਰਮਿ ਪਵੈ ਨੀਸਾਣੁ ॥

nadarī karam pavai nīsāṇ.

They receive the Mark of Grace from the Merciful Lord.

ਕਚ ਪਕਾਈ ਓਥੈ ਪਾਇ ॥

kach pakā-ī othai pā-i.

The ripe and the unripe, the good and the bad, shall there be judged.

ਨਾਨਕ ਗਇਆ ਜਾਪੈ ਜਾਇ ॥੩੪॥

nānak ga-i-ā jāpai jā-i. ‖34‖

O Nānak, when you go home, you will see this. ‖34‖

ਧਰਮ ਖੰਡ ਕਾ ਏਹੋ ਧਰਮੁ ॥

dharam khaṇḍ kā ayho dharam.

This is righteous living in the realm of Dharma.

ਗਿਆਨ ਖੰਡ ਕਾ ਆਖਹੁ ਕਰਮੁ ॥

gi-ān khaṇḍ kā ākhah(u) karam.

And now we speak of the realm of spiritual wisdom.

ਕੇਤੇ ਪਵਣ ਪਾਣੀ ਵੈਸੰਤਰ ਕੇਤੇ ਕਾਨ ਮਹੇਸ ॥

kaytay pavaṇ pāṇī vaisantar kaytay kān mahays.

So many winds, waters, and fires; so many Krishnas and Shivas.

ਕੇਤੇ ਬਰਮੇ ਘਾੜਤਿ ਘੜੀਅਹਿ ਰੂਪ ਰੰਗ ਕੇ ਵੇਸ ॥

kaytay baramay ghāṛat ghaṛī-ahi rūp rang kay vays.

*So many Brahmas, fashioning forms of great beauty,
adorned and dressed in many colors.*

ਕੇਤੀਆ ਕਰਮ ਭੂਮੀ ਮੇਰ ਕੇਤੇ ਕੇਤੇ ਧੂ ਉਪਦੇਸ ॥

kaytī-ā karam bhūmī mayr kaytay kaytay dhū upadays.

So many worlds and lands for working out karma.
So very many lessons to be learned!

ਕੇਤੇ ਇੰਦ ਚੰਦ ਸੂਰ ਕੇਤੇ ਕੇਤੇ ਮੰਡਲ ਦੇਸ ॥

kaytay ind chand sūr kaytay kaytay mandal days.

So many Indras, so many moons and suns, so many worlds and lands.

ਕੇਤੇ ਸਿਧ ਬੁਧ ਨਾਥ ਕੇਤੇ ਕੇਤੇ ਦੇਵੀ ਵੇਸ ॥

kaytay sidh budh nāth kaytay kaytay dayvī vays.

So many Siddhas and Buddhas, so many Yogic masters.
So many goddesses of various kinds.

ਕੇਤੇ ਦੇਵ ਦਾਨਵ ਮੁਨਿ ਕੇਤੇ ਕੇਤੇ ਰਤਨ ਸਮੁੰਦ ॥

kaytay dayv dānav mun kaytay kaytay ratan samund.

So many demi-gods and demons, so many silent sages. So many oceans of jewels.

ਕੇਤੀਆ ਖਾਣੀ ਕੇਤੀਆ ਬਾਣੀ ਕੇਤੇ ਪਾਤ ਨਰਿੰਦ ॥

kaytī-ā khānī kaytī-ā banī kaytay pāt narind.

So many ways of life, so many languages. So many dynasties of rulers.

ਕੇਤੀਆ ਸੁਰਤੀ ਸੇਵਕ ਕੇਤੇ ਨਾਨਕ ਅੰਤੁ ਨ ਅੰਤੁ ॥੩੫॥

kaytī-ā suratī sayvak kaytay nānak ant na ant. ‖ 35‖

So many intuitive people, so many selfless servants.
O Nānak, His limit has no limit! ‖35‖

ਗਿਆਨ ਖੰਡ ਮਹਿ ਗਿਆਨੁ ਪਰਚੰਡੁ ॥

gi-ān khand mah(i) gi-ān parachand.

In the realm of wisdom, spiritual wisdom reigns supreme.

ਤਿਥੈ ਨਾਦ ਬਿਨੋਦ ਕੋਡ ਅਨੰਦੁ ॥

tithai nād binod koḍ anand.

The Sound Current of the Naad vibrates there,
amidst the sounds and the sights of bliss.

ਸਰਮ ਖੰਡ ਕੀ ਬਾਣੀ ਰੂਪੁ ॥

saram khanḍ kī baṇī rūp.

In the realm of humility, the Word is Beauty.

ਤਿਥੈ ਘਾੜਤਿ ਘੜੀਐ ਬਹੁਤੁ ਅਨੂਪੁ ॥

tithai ghāṛat ghaṛī-ai bahut anūp.

Forms of incomparable beauty are fashioned there.

ਤਾ ਕੀਆ ਗਲਾ ਕਥੀਆ ਨਾ ਜਾਹਿ ॥

tā kī-ā galā kathī-ā nā jāh(i).

These things cannot be described.

ਜੇ ਕੋ ਕਹੈ ਪਿਛੈ ਪਛੁਤਾਇ ॥

jay ko kahai pichhai pachhutā-i.

One who tries to speak of these shall regret the attempt.

ਤਿਥੈ ਘੜੀਐ ਸੁਰਤਿ ਮਤਿ ਮਨਿ ਬੁਧਿ ॥

tithai ghaṛī-ai surat mat man budh.

The intuitive consciousness, intellect, and understanding
of the mind are shaped there.

ਤਿਥੈ ਘੜੀਐ ਸੁਰਾ ਸਿਧਾ ਕੀ ਸੁਧਿ ॥੩੬॥

tithai ghaṛī-ai surā sidhā kī sudh. ‖ 36‖

The consciousness of the spiritual warriors and the Siddhas,
the beings of spiritual perfection, are shaped there. ‖36‖

ਕਰਮ ਖੰਡ ਕੀ ਬਾਣੀ ਜੋਰੁ ॥

karam khand kī banī jor.

In the realm of karma, the Word is Power.

ਤਿਥੈ ਹੋਰੁ ਨ ਕੋਈ ਹੋਰੁ ॥

tithai hor na ko-ī hor.

No one else dwells there,

ਤਿਥੈ ਜੋਧ ਮਹਾਬਲ ਸੂਰ ॥

tithai jodh mahābal sūr.

except the warriors of great power, the spiritual heroes.

ਤਿਨ ਮਹਿ ਰਾਮੁ ਰਹਿਆ ਭਰਪੂਰ ॥

tin mah(i) rām rahi-ā bharapūr.

They are totally fulfilled, imbued with the Lord's Essence.

ਤਿਥੈ ਸੀਤੋ ਸੀਤਾ ਮਹਿਮਾ ਮਾਹਿ ॥

tithai sīto sītā mahimā māh(i).

Myriads of Sītas are there, cool and calm in their majestic glory.

ਤਾ ਕੇ ਰੂਪ ਨ ਕਥਨੇ ਜਾਹਿ ॥

tā kay rūp na kathanay jāh(i).

Their beauty cannot be described.

ਨਾ ਓਹਿ ਮਰਹਿ ਨ ਠਾਗੇ ਜਾਹਿ ॥

nā oh(i) marah(i) na thāgay jāh(i).

Neither death nor deception comes to those,

ਜਿਨ ਕੈ ਰਾਮੁ ਵਸੈ ਮਨ ਮਾਹਿ ॥

jin kai rām vasai man māh(i).

within whose minds the Lord abides.

ਤਿਥੈ ਭਗਤ ਵਸਹਿ ਕੇ ਲੋਅ ॥

tithai bhagat vasah(i) kay lo-a.

The devotees of many worlds dwell there.

ਕਰਹਿ ਅਨੰਦੁ ਸਚਾ ਮਨਿ ਸੋਇ ॥

karah(i) anand sachā man so-i.

They celebrate; their minds are imbued with the True Lord.

ਸਚ ਖੰਡਿ ਵਸੈ ਨਿਰੰਕਾਰੁ ॥

sach khanḍ vasai nirankār.

In the realm of Truth, the Formless Lord abides.

ਕਰਿ ਕਰਿ ਵੇਖੈ ਨਦਰਿ ਨਿਹਾਲ ॥

kar kar vaykhai nadar nihāl.

Having created the creation, He watches over it.
By His Glance of Grace, He bestows happiness.

ਤਿਥੈ ਖੰਡ ਮੰਡਲ ਵਰਭੰਡ ॥

tithai khanḍ manḍal varabhanḍ.

There are planets, solar systems, and galaxies.

ਜੇ ਕੋ ਕਥੈ ਤ ਅੰਤ ਨ ਅੰਤ ॥

jay ko kathai ta ant na ant.

If one speaks of them, there is no limit, no end.

ਤਿਥੈ ਲੋਅ ਲੋਅ ਆਕਾਰ ॥

tithai lo-a lo-a ākār.

There are worlds upon worlds of His Creation.

ਜਿਵ ਜਿਵ ਹੁਕਮੁ ਤਿਵੈ ਤਿਵ ਕਾਰ ॥

jiv jiv hukam tivai tiv kār.

As He commands, so they exist.

ਵੇਖੈ ਵਿਗਸੈ ਕਰਿ ਵੀਚਾਰੁ ॥

vaykhai vigasai kar vīchār.

He watches over all, and contemplating the creation, He rejoices.

ਨਾਨਕ ਕਥਨਾ ਕਰੜਾ ਸਾਰੁ ॥੩੭॥

nānak kathanā kararā sār. ||37||

O Nānak, to describe this is as hard as steel! ||37||

ਜਤੁ ਪਾਹਾਰਾ ਧੀਰਜੁ ਸੁਨਿਆਰੁ ॥

jat pāhārā dhīraj suni-ār.

Let self-control be the furnace, and patience the goldsmith.

ਅਹਰਣਿ ਮਤਿ ਵੇਦੁ ਹਥੀਆਰੁ ॥

aharan mat vayd hathī-ār.

Let understanding be the anvil, and spiritual wisdom the tools.

ਭਉ ਖਲਾ ਅਗਨਿ ਤਪ ਤਾਉ ॥

bha-u khalā agan tap tā-u.

With the Fear of God as the bellows, fan the flames of Tapa, the body's inner heat.

ਭਾਂਡਾ ਭਾਉ ਅੰਮ੍ਰਿਤੁ ਤਿਤੁ ਢਾਲਿ ॥

bhāndā bhā-u amrit tit dhāl.

In the crucible of love, melt the Nectar of the Name,

ਘੜੀਐ ਸਬਦੁ ਸਚੀ ਟਕਸਾਲ ॥

gharī-ai sabad sachī takasāl.

and mint the True Coin of the Shabad, the Word of God.

ਜਿਨ ਕਉ ਨਦਰਿ ਕਰਮੁ ਤਿਨ ਕਾਰ ॥

jin ka-u nadar karam tin kār.

Such is the karma of those upon whom He has cast His Glance of Grace.

ਨਾਨਕ ਨਦਰੀ ਨਦਰਿ ਨਿਹਾਲ ॥੩੮॥

nānak nadarī nadar nihāl. || 38||

O Nānak, the Merciful Lord, by His Grace, uplifts and exalts them. ||38||

ਸਲੋਕੁ ॥

salok.

Salok:

ਪਵਣੁ ਗੁਰੁ ਪਾਣੀ ਪਿਤਾ ਮਾਤਾ ਧਰਤਿ ਮਹਤੁ ॥

pavan gurū pāṇī pitā mātā dharat mahat.

Air is the Gurū, Water is the Father, and Earth is the Great Mother of all.

ਦਿਵਸੁ ਰਾਤਿ ਦੁਇ ਦਾਈ ਦਾਇਆ ਖੇਲੈ ਸਗਲ ਜਗਤੁ ॥

divas rāt du-i dā-ī dā-i-ā khaylai sagal jagat.

Day and night are the two nurses, in whose lap all the world is at play.

ਚੰਗਿਆਈਆ ਬੁਰਿਆਈਆ ਵਾਚੈ ਧਰਮੁ ਹਦੂਰਿ ॥

changi-ā-ī-ā buri-ā-ī-ā vāchai dharam hadūr.

*Good deeds and bad deeds—the record is read out
in the Presence of the Lord of Dharma.*

ਕਰਮੀ ਆਪੋ ਆਪਣੀ ਕੇ ਨੇੜੈ ਕੇ ਦੂਰਿ ॥

karamī āpo āpaṇī kay nayṛai kay dūr.

*According to their own actions, some are drawn closer,
and some are driven farther away.*

ਜਿਨੀ ਨਾਮੁ ਧਿਆਇਆ ਗਏ ਮਸਕਤਿ ਘਾਲਿ ॥

jinī nām dhi-ā-i-ā ga-ay masakat ghāl.

*Those who have meditated on the Nām, the Name of the Lord,
and departed after having worked by the sweat of their brows,*

ਨਾਨਕ ਤੇ ਮੁਖ ਉਜਲੇ ਕੇਤੀ ਛੁਟੀ ਨਾਲਿ ॥੧॥

nānak tay mukh ujalay kaytī chhuṭī nāl. || 1||

O Nānak, their faces are radiant in the Court of the Lord,
and many are saved along with them! || 1||

ਵਾਹਿਗੁਰੂ ਜੀ ਕਾ ਖਾਲਸਾ, ਵਾਹਿਗੁਰੂ ਜੀ ਕੀ ਫਤਹਿ!

Wāhegurū jī kā Khālsā ! Wāhegurū jī kī Fateh!

The Khālsā (those who live in purity) belong to God, Victory belongs to God!

~ *Appendix B* ~

KUNDALINI YOGA SETS[1]

SŪRYA NAMASKĀRA — SUN SALUTATIONS

1. **Standing Straight.** Stand up straight, feet together, toes and heels touching, weight evenly distributed between both feet. Find your balance. Hold your arms by your sides, fingers together. Eyes gaze straight ahead (Figure Sun-1).

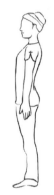

Figure Sun-1

2. **Stretching Up.** Inhale. Bring your arms up over your head, palms touching. Elongate your spine, lifting the chest and relaxing your shoulders. Be sure not to compress the vertebrae of the neck and lower back. Look up at the thumbs (Figure Sun-2).

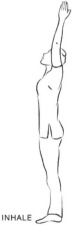

INHALE

Figure Sun-2

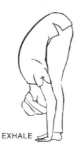

EXHALE

Figure Sun-3

3. Front Bend. Exhale and bend your torso forward. As you bend, keep your spine straight, elongating it as if reaching forward with the top of the head. When you can no longer hold your spine straight, relax the head as close to the knees as possible. Ideally, touch your chin to the shins. Keep your knees straight and place hands on the floor on either side of the feet, with fingertips and tips of the toes in line. Gaze at the tip of the nose (Figure Sun-3).

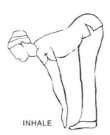

INHALE

Figure Sun-4

4. Inhale, raise your head up, straighten the spine, keeping the hands or fingertips on the floor. Gaze at the Third Eye Point (Figure Sun-4).

5. Push-Up. Exhale and bend your knees, stepping or jumping back so that the legs are straight out behind you, balancing on the bottoms of the bent toes. Elbows are bent, hugging the rib cage, and palms are flat on the floor under the shoulders, with fingers spread wide apart. The body is in a straight line from forehead to ankles. Keep yourself equally balanced between hands and feet. Do not push forward with your toes (Figure Sun-5).

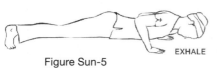

EXHALE

Figure Sun-5

6. **Cobra Pose.** From this
   position, inhale, straighten
   your elbows, and arch the
   back. Stretch through the
   upper back so that there is
   no pressure on the lower
   spine. Point your forehead
   to the sky and gaze at the tip of your
   nose. Spread your fingers wide apart
   (Figure Sun-6).

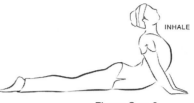

Figure Sun-6

7. **Triangle Pose.** Exhale and
   lift your hips up so that the
   body balances in an inverted
   V shape. Feet and palms are
   flat on the floor, elbows and
   knees straight. Spread your
   fingers wide apart. Gaze
   toward your navel and hold this
   position for five breaths. So as not
   to bend the head, I recommend an
   inner gaze toward the navel with the
   eyes closed (Figure Sun-7).

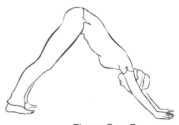

Figure Sun-7

8. Inhale and jump or step back into
   position 4 (Figure Sun-8). Gaze at
   the Third Eye Point.

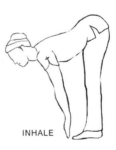

Figure Sun-8

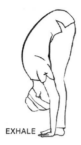

EXHALE

Figure Sun-9

9. **Front Bend.** Exhale and bend forward into position 3 (Figure Sun-9). Gaze at the tip of the nose.

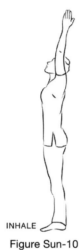

INHALE

Figure Sun-10

10. **Stretching Up.** Inhale and come all the way up into position 2 (Figure Sun-10). Look up at the thumbs.

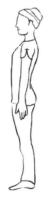

Figure Sun-11

11. **Standing Straight.** Exhale and return to the starting position with arms by your sides, eyes gazing forward (Figure Sun-11).

BASIC SPINAL ENERGY SERIES

For the following exercises that ask for 108 repetitions, you have the option to do them twenty-four times when you're just starting out. If you do this, extend the rest periods from one to two minutes. Similarly, if you can't sit on the floor, feel free to use a chair with both of your feet flat on the ground, your sitz bones balanced on the seat to keep your spine in a balanced position.

1. **Spinal Flex.** Sit in Easy Pose (page 98). Grab your ankles with both hands and deeply inhale. Flex the spine forward and lift the chest up (Figure Spine-1a). When you exhale, flex the spine backward (Figure Spine-1b). Keep the head level so it does not wobble around. Repeat 108 times. Rest for one minute in Easy Pose with your eyes closed.

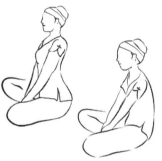

Figures Spine-1a & 1b

2. **Spinal Flex.** Sit on your heels. Place your hands flat on the thighs. Flex your spine forward with the inhale (Figure Spine-2a) and backward with the exhale (Figure Spine-2b). Mentally vibrate the syllable "sat" on the inhale and "nām" on the exhale. Repeat 108 times. Rest for two minutes while sitting on your heels with your eyes closed.

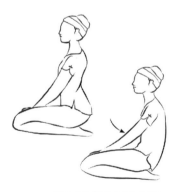

Figures Spine-2a & 2b

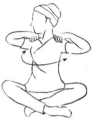

Figure Spine-3

3. **Spinal Twist.** In Easy Pose, grasp the shoulders with fingers in front, thumbs in back. Inhale and twist to your left, exhale and twist to your right (Figure Spine-3). Take long, deep breaths. Continue twenty-six times and inhale, facing forward. Rest one minute in Easy Pose with your eyes closed.

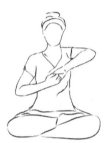

Figure Spine-4

4. **Bear Grip.** Lock your fingers in Bear Grip at the heart center (Figure Spine-4). Move your elbows in a seesaw motion, breathing long and deep with the movement. Continue twenty-six times, inhale, exhale, and pull on the lock. Relax for thirty seconds.

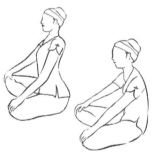

Figures Spine-5a & 5b

5. **Spinal Flex.** In Easy Pose, grasp the knees firmly and begin to flex the upper spine while you keep your elbows straight. Inhale forward (Figure Spine-5a), exhale back (Figure Spine-5b). Repeat 108 times. Rest for one minute in Easy Pose with your eyes closed.

6. **Shoulder Shrugs.** Shrug both shoulders up when you inhale (Figure Spine-6) and down when you exhale. Do this for two minutes, but not more. Inhale and hold fifteen seconds with shoulders pressed up. Relax your shoulders.

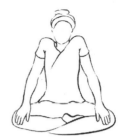

Figure Spine-6

7. **Neck Rolls.** Roll the neck slowly to the right five times, then to the left five times (Figure Spine-7). Inhale and straighten the neck.

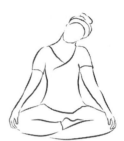

Figure Spine-7

8. **Bear Grip.** Lock your fingers in Bear Grip at the throat level (Figure Spine-8a). Inhale and apply Mūlbandh (page 94). Exhale and do the same. Then raise your hands above the top of your head (Figure Spine-8b). Inhale and apply Mūlbandh, then exhale and apply Mūlbandh again. Repeat the cycle two more times. As you work with holding your breath, I recommend beginning with ten seconds and increasing as you become able.

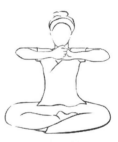

Figure Spine-8a

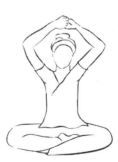

Figure Spine-8b

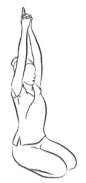

Figure Spine-9a

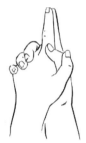

Figure Spine-9b

9. **Sat Kriya.** Sit on your heels with arms stretched over the head and palms together. Interlace your fingers except for the two index fingers, which point straight up (Figure Spine-9a). Men cross the right thumb over the left thumb; women cross the left thumb over the right (Figure Spine-9b). Chant "sat" and pull your navel point in; chant "nām" and relax it. Continue powerfully with a steady rhythm for at least three minutes, then inhale, apply Mūlbandh, and squeeze the energy from the base of your spine to the top of the skull. Exhale, hold the breath out, and apply all the locks (Neck, Diaphragm, and Mūlbandh [page 94]). Inhale and relax. As you increase the length of time you practice Sat Kriya, your rest period should be at least twice as long as the amount of time that you do Sat Kriya.

10. **Relax.** Relax completely on your back for fifteen minutes. When you finish, practice the Coming Out of Relaxation Exercises as described in chapter 6 (page 92).

AWAKENING TO YOUR TEN BODIES

As a reminder, the ten bodies these poses awaken are Soul Body, Negative Mind, Positive Mind, Neutral Mind, Physical Body, Arcline, Auric Body, Prānic Body, Subtle Body, and Radiant Body.

1. **Stretch Pose.** Lie on your back with arms at your sides. Raise your head and your legs six inches. Raise the hands six inches with palms facing each other slightly over the hips to build energy across the Navel Point. Point your toes, keep your eyes focused on the tips of the toes, and do Breath of Fire (page 94). Perform this pose from one to three minutes (Figure Ten Bodies-1).

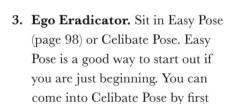

Figure Ten Bodies-1

2. **Nose to Knees.** Bring the knees to your chest, with arms wrapped around knees. Tuck your nose between the knees and begin Breath of Fire. Perform this pose from one to three minutes (Figure Ten Bodies-2).

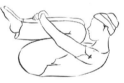

Figure Ten Bodies-2

3. **Ego Eradicator.** Sit in Easy Pose (page 98) or Celibate Pose. Easy Pose is a good way to start out if you are just beginning. You can come into Celibate Pose by first

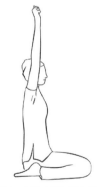

Figure Ten Bodies-3a

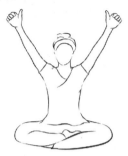

Figure Ten Bodies-3b

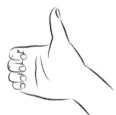

Figure Ten Bodies-3c

sitting on the heels. Then spread the feet apart so that you can place your buttocks on the ground, with your feet on either side of the hips (Figure Ten Bodies-3a). Raise the arms to a sixty-degree angle (Figure Ten Bodies-3b). Curl your fingertips onto the pads at the base of the fingers (Figure Ten Bodies-3c). Plug your thumbs into the sky. With eyes closed, concentrate above your head, and do Breath of Fire. Perform this pose from one to three minutes. To end, inhale and touch the thumb-tips together overhead. Exhale and apply Mūlbandh (page 94). Inhale and relax.

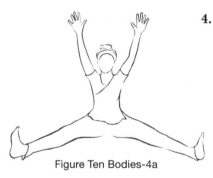

Figure Ten Bodies-4a

4. **Life Nerve Stretch.** Sit with legs stretched wide apart. With arms overhead, inhale (Figure Ten Bodies-4a). Then exhale, stretch down, and grab the toes of your left foot (Figure Ten Bodies-4b). Inhale, come straight up, then exhale and stretch down over the right leg and grab your toes. Repeat for one to three minutes.

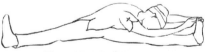

Figure Ten Bodies-4b

5. **Life Nerve Stretch (Center).**
Continue to sit with legs
stretched wide apart. Hold
onto the toes of both feet
(Figure Ten Bodies-5a), exhale
as you stretch down, bringing
your forehead toward the floor
(Figure Ten Bodies-5b), and inhale
as you sit up. Continue for one
to three minutes.

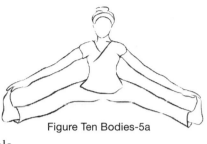

Figure Ten Bodies-5a

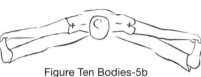

Figure Ten Bodies-5b

6. **Spinal Flex (Camel Ride).** Sit in
Easy Pose. Grab your shins in front
with both hands. Inhale. Flex your
spine forward and rock forward on
buttocks (Figure Ten Bodies-6a).
Then exhale, flex the spine
backward, and roll back on your
buttocks (Figure Ten Bodies-6b).
Keep the head level and arms fairly
straight and relaxed. Repeat for one
to three minutes.

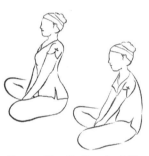

Figures Ten Bodies-6a & 6b

7. **Spinal Flex on Heels.** Sit on
your heels. Place hands flat
on your thighs. Flex the spine
forward on the inhale (Figure
Ten Bodies-7a), backward on the
exhale (Figure Ten Bodies-7b).
Focus at the Third Eye Point.
Repeat for one to three minutes.

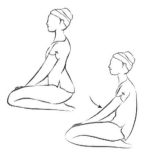

Figures Ten Bodies-7a & 7b

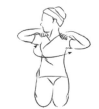

Figure Ten Bodies-8

8. Spinal Twist. Still on the heels, grasp your shoulders with the fingers in front, thumbs in back. Inhale and twist to the left, exhale and twist to the right (do not reverse this order) (Figure Ten Bodies-8). Keep your elbows high and parallel to the floor. Continue for one to three minutes.

Figure Ten Bodies-9

9. Elbow Lifts. Grasp your shoulders as in the previous exercise. Inhale and raise your elbows up so the backs of your wrists touch behind your neck (Figure Ten Bodies-9). Exhale and lower the elbows to shoulder height, and repeat for one to three minutes.

Figure Ten Bodies-10a

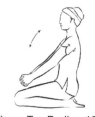

Figure Ten Bodies-10b

10. Arm Pumps. Sitting on your heels, interlace your fingers in Venus Lock as follows: If you are a woman, place the palms together, interlace the fingers with the right pinky on the bottom closest to the ground, and cross the thumbs with the left thumb over the right thumb. The tip of the left thumb presses the fleshy mound at the base of the right thumb (Figure Ten Bodies-10a). Reverse the sequence if you are a man. With elbows straight (Figure Ten Bodies-10b), inhale and stretch your arms up over your head (Figure Ten Bodies-10c), then exhale and bring the hands back to your lap. Repeat for one to three minutes.

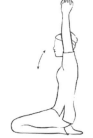

Figure Ten Bodies-10c

11. **Alternate Shoulder Shrugs.** Sit in Easy Pose with hands resting on your knees. Inhale and shrug your left shoulder up (Figure Ten Bodies-11). Exhale and raise your right shoulder up as you lower the left shoulder. Continue for one minute. Then reverse the breath so you inhale as you shrug your right shoulder up and exhale as you shrug your left shoulder up and lower the right shoulder. Continue for one minute.

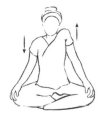

Figure Ten Bodies-11

12. **Shoulder Shrugs.** Inhale and shrug both shoulders up (Figure Ten Bodies-12), exhale down. Continue for one minute.

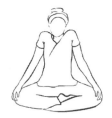

Figure Ten Bodies-12

13. **Neck Turns.** Remain sitting in Easy Pose, hands on knees. Inhale and twist your head to the left; exhale and twist it to the right (Figure Ten Bodies-13), as if you were slowly shaking your head no. Continue for one minute. Then reverse your breath, so that you inhale and twist to the right and exhale and twist to the left. Continue for one minute. Inhale deeply, concentrate at the Third Eye Point, and slowly exhale.

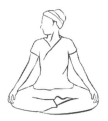

Figure Ten Bodies-13

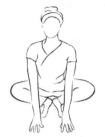

Figure Ten Bodies-14a

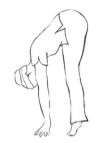

Figure Ten Bodies-14b

14. **Frog Pose.** Squat down so your buttocks are on your heels. The heels should touch and be off the ground. Put your fingertips on the ground between your knees. Keep your head up (Figure Ten Bodies-14a). Inhale, straighten your legs, lifting your hips and keeping the fingers on the ground (Figure Ten Bodies-14b). Exhale and come back to squatting down, face forward. Your inhalations and exhalations should be strong. Continue this cycle fifty-four times.

15. **Relaxation.** Deeply relax on your back. Relax for five to eleven minutes. Afterward, practice the Coming Out of Relaxation Exercises as described in chapter 6 (page 92).

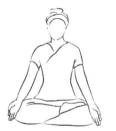

Figure Ten Bodies-16

16. **Laya Yoga Meditation.** With the breath, visualize the sound spiraling up in a counterclockwise manner from the base of the spine to the top of your head in three and a half circles in a helix format. Close the eyes and concentrate at the Third Eye Point. As the

sound spirals up to the top, feel
it emanating out through the
tenth gate at the top of the head
at the last half circle. Sit in Easy
Pose with hands on knees in Giān
Mudra (thumb and index finger
together) (Figure Ten Bodies-16).
Chant "ek ong kār(uh), satinām(uh)
sirī, wā(uh) hegurū." On "ek" pull
the navel. On each final "uh," lift
the diaphragm up firmly. The
"uh" sound is more of a powerful
movement of the diaphragm than
a purposefully projected sound.
Relax the navel and abdomen on
"hegurū." Continue for eleven to
thirty-one minutes.

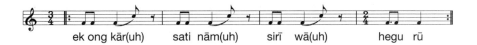

ek ong kār(uh)   sati nām(uh)   sirī   wā(uh)   hegu rū

Musical Notation for Laya Yoga Meditation

KRIYA FOR ELEVATION

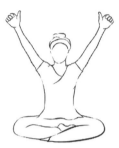

Figure Elevation-1a

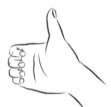

Figure Elevation-1b

1. **Ego Eradicator.** Sit in Easy Pose (page 98). Raise your arms to a sixty-degree angle (Figure Elevation-1a). Curl your fingertips onto the pads at the base of the fingers (Figure Elevation-1b). Plug the thumbs into the sky. Eyes closed, concentrate above your head, and do Breath of Fire (page 94) for one to three minutes. To end, inhale and touch the thumb tips together overhead. Exhale and apply Mūlbandh (page 94). Inhale and relax.

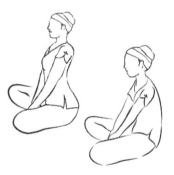

Figures Elevation-2a & 2b

2. **Spinal Flex.** Sitting in Easy Pose, grasp your shins with both hands. As you inhale, flex the spine forward and lift your chest (Figure Elevation-2a). As you exhale, flex the spine back, keeping your shoulders relaxed and head straight (Figure Elevation-2b). Continue rhythmically with deep breaths for one to three minutes. To end: inhale, exhale, and relax.

3. **Spinal Twist.** In Easy Pose, grab your shoulders, with the thumbs in back and fingers in front. Keep the elbows high, with arms parallel to the ground. Inhale as you twist your head and torso to the left. Exhale as you twist to the right (Figure Elevation-3). Continue for one to four minutes. To end, inhale while facing straight forward. Exhale and relax.

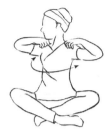

Figure Elevation-3

4. **Front Life Nerve Stretch.** Stretch both legs straight out in front. Grab your toes in finger lock (index finger and middle finger pull the toe, and the thumb presses the nail of the big toe) (Figure Elevation-4a). Exhale as you lengthen the core of the spine, bending forward from the navel, continuing to lengthen your spine. The head follows last (Figure Elevation-4b). Inhale and use your legs to push up. The head comes up last. Continue to fold forward on the exhale and rise up on the inhale with deep, powerful breathing for one to three minutes. Inhale up and hold the breath briefly. Stay up and exhale completely, holding the breath out for just a moment. Inhale and relax.

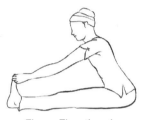

Figure Elevation-4a

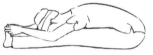

Figure Elevation-4b

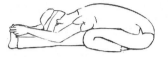

Figure Elevation-5

5. **Modified Maha Mudra.** Sit with your right heel tucked into the perineum and your left leg extended forward. Grasp the big toe of your left foot with both hands, applying pressure against the toenail. Pull Neck Lock (page 94). Exhale and bring your elbows toward the ground as you lengthen the spine, bending forward from your navel, continuing to lengthen the spine, bringing your head toward your knee, the spine staying straight (Figure Elevation-5). Hold, with Breath of Fire (page 94) for one to two minutes. Inhale. Exhale and stretch the head and torso forward and down. Hold the breath out briefly. Inhale, switch legs, and repeat the exercise. Relax.

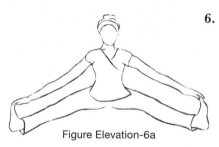

Figure Elevation-6a

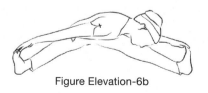

Figure Elevation-6b

6. **Life Nerve Stretch.** Spread your legs wide and grasp your toes. Inhale and stretch the spine straight, pulling back on your toes (Figure Elevation-6a). Exhale and, bending at the waist, bring your head down to the left knee. Inhale up in the center position and exhale down, bringing the head to your right knee (Figure Elevation-6b). Continue, with powerful breathing for one to two minutes. Then inhale up in the center position and exhale, bending straight forward from

the waist, touching your forehead to the floor (Figure Elevation-6c). Continue this up and down motion for one minute, then inhale up, stretching the spine straight. Exhale while bringing your forehead to the floor. Hold the breath out briefly as you stretch forward and down. Inhale and relax.

Figure Elevation-6c

7. **Cobra Pose.** Lie on your stomach with palms flat on the floor under your shoulders. Keep your heels together with the soles of the feet facing up. Inhale into Cobra Pose, arching the spine, vertebra by vertebra, from neck to the base of the spine until your arms are straight (Figure Elevation-7). Begin Breath of Fire. Continue for one to three minutes. Then inhale, arching the spine as far as you can. Exhale, hold the breath out briefly, and apply Mūlbandh. Inhale. Exhaling slowly, bend the elbows to lower your torso and relax the spine, vertebra by vertebra, from the base of the spine to the top. Relax, lying on the stomach with your chin on the floor, and arms to the sides.

Figure Elevation-7

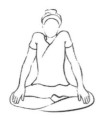

Figure Elevation-8

8. Shoulder Shrugs. Sit in Easy Pose. Place hands on the knees. Inhale and shrug your shoulders up toward the ears (Figure Elevation-8). Exhale and drop the shoulders down. Continue rhythmically with powerful breathing for one to two minutes. Inhale. Exhale and relax.

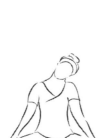

Figure Elevation-9

9. Neck Rolls. Sit in Easy Pose. Begin rolling your neck clockwise in a circular motion, bringing the right ear toward the right shoulder, the back of the head toward the back of the neck, the left ear toward the left shoulder, and the chin toward the chest. Keep your shoulders relaxed and motionless. Let your neck gently stretch as the head circles around (Figure Elevation-9). Continue for one to two minutes. Reverse the direction of the neck rolls and continue for one to two minutes more. Bring your head to a central position and relax.

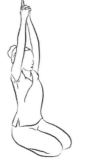

Figure Elevation-10a

10. Sat Kriya. Sit on your heels with arms overhead and palms together. Interlace your fingers except for the index fingers, which point straight up (Figure Elevation-10a). Men cross the right thumb over the left thumb; women cross the left thumb over the right (Figure Elevation-10b). Begin to chant "sat nām" emphatically

in a constant rhythm about eight
times per ten seconds. Chant "sat"
from the navel point and solar
plexus, and pull the navel all the
way in and up. On "nām," relax the
navel. Continue for three to seven
minutes, then inhale and squeeze
the muscles tight from your buttocks
all the way up the back past your
shoulders. Mentally allow the energy
to flow through the top of your
skull. Exhale. Inhale deeply. Exhale
completely and apply the Mūlbandh
with breath held out. Inhale and
relax. This Kriya circulates the
Kundalini energy through the cycle
of the Chakras, aids in digestion,
and strengthens the nervous system.

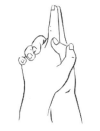

Figure Elevation-10b

11. **Relaxation.** Relax in Easy Pose or
on your back with arms at your sides,
palms up. Relaxation allows you to
enjoy and consciously integrate the
mind-body changes enacted by this
Kriya. It allows you to sense the
extension of the self through the
magnetic field and the Aura and
allows the physical body to deeply
relax. Suggested relaxation time is
eleven to fifteen minutes; make sure
you relax for at least twice as long
as your Sat Kriya practice. If you
have relaxed on your back, practice
the Coming Out of Relaxation
Exercises as described in chapter 6
(page 92).

KRIYA FOR MORNING SĀDHANĀ

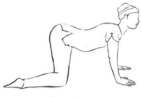

Cow Pose
Figure Morning-1a

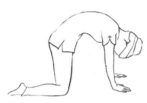

Cat Pose
Figure Morning-1b

1. **Cat-Cow.** Come into a position supporting your body on your hands and knees, with knees shoulder-width apart, heels touching behind, and arms straight. Do not bend your elbows. Inhale and flex the spine downward as if someone were sitting on your back. Stretch your neck and head back. This is Cow Pose (Figure Morning-1a). Then exhale and flex the spine up, bringing your chin toward the chest into Cat Pose (Figure Morning-1b). Continue rhythmically with powerful breathing for three minutes. Gradually increase your speed as you feel the spine becoming more flexible. Inhale in the original position. Exhale and relax. Then inhale into Cow Pose and hold for ten seconds. Exhale and relax.

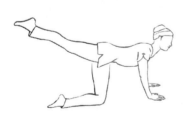

Figure Morning-2a

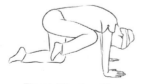

Figure Morning-2b

2. **Cow Pose Variation.** In Cow Pose, inhale and raise your right leg and head up as high as possible (Figure Morning-2a). Exhale and swing your knee under the body, and bring your head down (Figure Morning-2b). Do thirty repetitions, then inhale and lift your right leg up. Exhale and hold your breath for ten seconds. Inhale and repeat with left leg. Do thirty repetitions.

3. **Hugging Spinal Bend.** Sit on your heels with knees spread apart. Grasp opposite arms just above the elbows, letting arms rest against your chest. Bend from side to side in a smooth motion. Inhale center, exhale to each side (Figure Morning-3). Continue for one minute. Inhale, hold, and exhale.

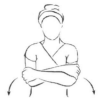

Figure Morning-3

4. **Spinal Twist Variation with Giān Mudra.** Sitting on your heels, raise your arms with the elbows bent at ninety degrees and the upper arms parallel to the floor. With hands in Giān Mudra, focus at the Third Eye Point, and twist your torso, inhaling left, exhaling right with powerful breath (Figure Morning-4). Continue for sixty repetitions. Inhale center, hold the breath, and focus. Exhale. Relax.

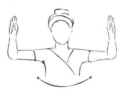

Figure Morning-4

5. **Spinal Flex.** Bring your knees together and place your hands palms down on thighs. Focus at the Third Eye Point, and flex your spine in rhythm with powerful breaths (Figure Morning-5). Do 108 flexes, then inhale, pull the locks, and hold for ten seconds. Exhale and sit still. Meditate silently on the breath, inhaling "sat," exhaling "nām," for thirty seconds. Inhale, exhale, and relax.

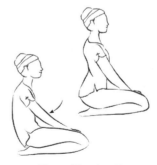

Figure Morning-5

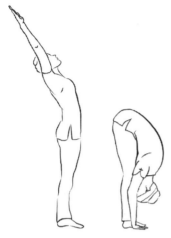

Figures Morning-6a & 6b

6. Front Bend. Stand up carefully and shake out your legs. Stand with feet shoulder-width apart. Hook your thumbs together. Inhale, raise arms over the head with arms hugging the ears. Stretch back, stretching the ribcage and using your full lung capacity. Relax your head back (Figure Morning-6a). Exhale forward and bend down, touching the floor, keeping your knees straight (Figure Morning-6b). Repeat thirty times. Inhale back and hold the stretch a few seconds. Exhale and bend forward at the waist. Let your arms hang down and completely relax for thirty seconds.

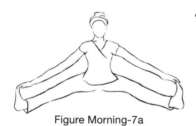

Figure Morning-7a

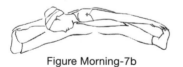

Figure Morning-7b

7. Life Nerve Stretch. Sit with your legs extended and spread apart. Reach down and grab your toes (Figure Morning-7a). Begin stretching, inhaling up to the center, exhaling down to the left. Then inhale up to the center, exhale down to the right (Figure Morning-7b). Continue for two minutes. Keep your knees straight, spread your legs further apart, and continue for one.

8. **Life Nerve Stretch.** In the same position as figure Morning-7a above, legs wide, continue: inhale up to the center, hold for three seconds, then exhale down to the center (Figure Morning-8), then begin stretching down in the center with continuous pressure and long, deep breaths for one minute. Inhale and stretch down a bit further. Exhale and come up.

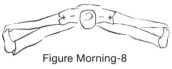

Figure Morning-8

9. **Butterfly.** Bring the soles of your feet together and clasp your fingers around your feet. Keep spine and head straight and begin bouncing the knees up and down. Let the knees move up and down vigorously, between ten and twelve inches, for one minute (Figures Morning-9a and Morning-9b).

Figure Morning-9a

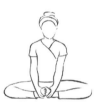

Figure Morning-9b

10. **Butterfly Bend.** Hold the same posture, keeping your knees pressed down. Stretch the spine up straight (Figure Morning-10a). Inhale up, exhale, and bend forward from the waist, bringing the torso down as far as you can (Figure Morning-10b). Continue, breathing powerfully for one minute. Inhale up, hold five seconds, exhale, stretch down, and hold for five seconds. Relax on your back.

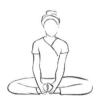

Figure Morning-10a

Figure Morning-10b

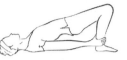

Figure Morning-11

11. Pelvic Lift. Still on your back, bend your knees, place your feet flat on the floor near the buttocks, and grab your ankles. Inhale and lift the hips as high as you can (Figure Morning-11), exhale, and lower them down. Inhale up, exhale down twenty-four times. To end, inhale, stretch up, and hold the breath ten seconds. Relax down and extend the legs straight out.

Figure Morning-12

12. Leg Lifts with Piston Motion. Lie on your back and point your toes. Lift both legs up eighteen inches. Inhale and draw the left knee to your chest. Exhale as you extend the left leg and simultaneously draw the right knee to your chest, keeping the lower leg parallel to the floor (Figure Morning-12). Continue this push-pull motion with powerful breathing for two minutes. Inhale and hold the legs up, extended out for ten seconds. Exhale and relax on the back.

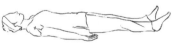

Figure Morning-13

13. Corpse Pose. Relax completely on your back for one minute (Figure Morning-13). Consciously circulate the energy from the navel point all through your body.

14. **Back Rolls.** Bring your knees to your chest, wrap your arms around them, and begin rocking on the spine forward and back (Figure Morning-14). Massage the whole spine for one to two minutes. Then rock up, turn around, and lie down on your stomach.

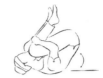

Figure Morning-14

15. **Cobra Pose.** Stretch up into Cobra Pose (Figure Morning-15). Relax your lower back and buttocks. Focus at the Third Eye Point and do Breath of Fire (page 94) for three minutes. Inhale, open your eyes, twist left, and look at your heels over your left shoulder. Hold fifteen seconds. Exhale center. Inhale, twist right, and look at your heels over your right shoulder. Hold fifteen seconds. Exhale center. Repeat one time. Inhale center, stretch up and back, and hold fifteen seconds. Exhale. Relax down.

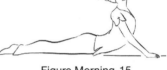

Figure Morning-15

16. **Yoga Mudra.** Carefully move into Yoga Mudra by sitting on your heels and bringing your forehead to the floor. Interlace your fingers behind your back and stretch your arms up (Figure Morning-16). Begin long, deep breathing. Draw the energy into the your upper back. Hold for one minute. Inhale, hold, exhale. Relax.

Figure Morning-16

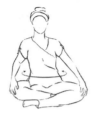

Figure Morning-17

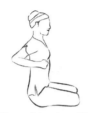

Figure Morning-18a

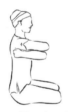

Figure Morning-18b

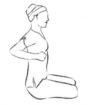

Figure Morning-18c

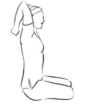

Figure Morning-18d

17. **Sufi Grind.** Sitting in Easy Pose (page 98), hold your kneecaps with your hands. Rotate the middle of your body in circles while keeping the head nearly still. Create a pressure at the base of the spine like a grinding wheel, using your arms for leverage (Figure Morning-17). Do this for one minute. Reverse direction and continue for another minute.

18. **Arm Swings.** Sit in Easy Pose. Inhale and draw elbows back by the sides of your rib cage (Figure Morning-18a). Exhale and swing your arms across the chest (Figure Morning-18b). Inhale again and draw the elbows back by the sides of your rib cage (Figure Morning-18c). Exhale and swing the arms up and back over your head (Figure Morning-18d). Repeat with a powerful breath and powerful motion for one to two minutes. Inhale, draw the elbows back, and stretch the chest forward. Hold for ten seconds. Relax.

19. **Shoulder Shrugs.** Sit with the spine straight and hands on knees with elbows relaxed. Inhale and squeeze your shoulders up (Figure Morning-19), exhale and drop them down, using a powerful breath. Do this 108 times.

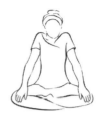

Figure Morning-19

20. **Neck Rolls.** Gently circle your head, breathing slowly and deeply, keeping the shoulders relaxed (Figure Morning-20). Do this for one minute, change directions for another minute.

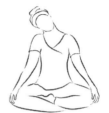

Figure Morning-20

21. **Arm Pumps with Venus Lock.** Sit on your heels and focus at the Third Eye Point. Join your hands in Venus Lock, as follows: If you are a woman, place the palms together, interlace the fingers with the right pinky on the bottom closest to the ground, and cross the thumbs with the left thumb over the right thumb. The tip of the left thumb presses the fleshy mound at the base of the right thumb (Figure Morning-21a). Reverse the sequence if you are a man. With elbows straight (Figure Morning-21b), inhale and bring the arms up sixty degrees above horizontal (Figure Morning-21c). Exhale and bring your arms sixty degrees below horizontal. Continue

Figure Morning-21a

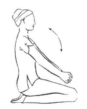

Figure Morning-21b

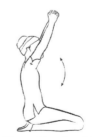

Figure Morning-21c

inhaling up and exhaling down powerfully. Do this seventy times.

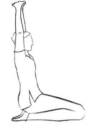

Figure Morning-22

22. **Arm Stretch with Interlaced Fingers.** Still sitting on your heels, bring your arms up overhead. Flip your hands over so the fingers interlace with palms facing up (Figure Morning-22). Roll your eyes up to the Tenth Gate and focus up above the head. Begin powerful Breath of Fire for one minute, then inhale and hold. Focus at the top of your skull at the Tenth Gate. Hold for fifteen seconds. Relax, exhale, and carefully bring your arms down.

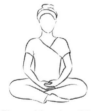

Figure Morning-23

23. **Meditate.** Come into Easy Pose and sit with a straight spine, one hand on top of the other in your lap, palms up (Figure Morning-23). Meditate silently, inhaling "sat" and exhaling "nām." Sit completely still and consciously expand your Aura. Focus deeply. Do this for one minute, then inhale, exhale, and relax.

Note: After practicing this Kriya, I recommend that you relax for five to eleven minutes on your back. After this, practice the Coming Out of Relaxation Exercises as described in chapter 6 (page 92).

MAGNETIC FIELD AND HEART CENTER

1. **Heart Center Opener.** Sit in Easy
   Pose (page 98). Hold the arms up
   at a sixty-degree angle with wrists
   and elbows straight, palms facing
   up (Figure Heart-1). Begin Breath
   of Fire (page 94) for one minute.
   Then inhale, hold the breath, and
   pump your stomach in and out
   sixteen times. Exhale and relax
   the breath. Continue the cycle for
   two to three minutes.

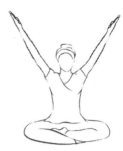

Figure Heart-1

2. Immediately sit on your heels with
   arms parallel to the ground at your
   sides. Let your hands hang limp from
   the wrists (Figure Heart-2). Begin
   Breath of Fire for three minutes.
   Inhale, hold, exhale, and relax.

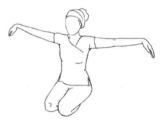

Figure Heart-2

3. **Stomach Pumps.** Sit on your heels.
   Spread your knees wide apart and
   lean back sixty degrees from the
   ground. Support your body with
   your arms straight down in back
   (Figure Heart-3a). Tilt your neck
   back, inhale, hold the breath, and
   pump your stomach in and out until
   you can no longer hold the breath.
   Exhale. Continue for one to two
   minutes. Tilt your spine back farther

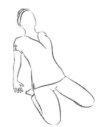

Figure Heart-3a

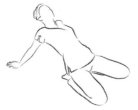

Figure Heart-3b

to thirty degrees (Figure Heart-3b) and continue the breathing cycle for another one to two minutes.

4. **Ong Sohung.** Still sitting on the heels with knees spread, put your forehead on the ground with arms stretched forward and relaxed in what is called Gurpranām (Figure Heart-4). Keep the posture and, after one minute, begin long, deep breathing for two minutes. Then chant the following Mantra in a call-and-response format for two minutes:
Teacher: Ong, Ong, Ong, Ong
Student: Ong, Ong, Ong, Ong
Teacher: Sohang, Sohang, Sohang, Sohang
Student: Sohang, Sohang, Sohang, Sohang

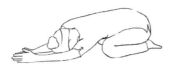

Figure Heart-4

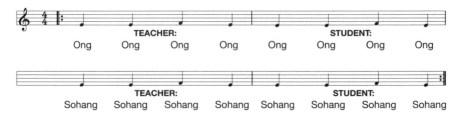

Ong Sohang Mantra

If practicing this set by yourself, hear a teacher's voice resonating the words silently, and then respond as the student.

5. **Life Nerve Stretch.** Grab your toes
   with legs slightly spread. Inhale,
   exhale, and reach down as you
   lengthen the core of your spine,
   bending forward from the navel,
   the head coming down last (Figure
   Heart-5). Hold for one minute.

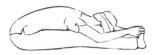

Figure Heart-5

6. **Back Platform.** Keep your
   body straight with heels on the
   ground and upper portion of
   your body held up by straight
   arms (Figure Heart-6a). Drop
   your head back and begin
   Breath of Fire. Do this for
   thirty seconds. **Back Platform
   Walk.** Begin to "walk" with
   legs growing progressively
   wider apart (Figure Heart-6b).
   Walk legs back together again
   and continue "walking" while
   doing Breath of Fire (page
   94). Maintain this for thirty
   seconds. Inhale, exhale, and move
   immediately into a front stretch
   holding the toes (Figure Heart-6c).
   Do this for one minute. Relax on
   the back for three minutes.

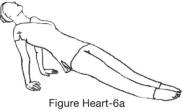

Figure Heart-6a

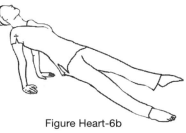

Figure Heart-6b

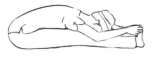

Figure Heart-6c

7. **Maha Mudra.** Sit on your left heel
   and stretch the right leg forward.
   Grab the right big toe with the right
   middle and index fingers, thumb
   pressing the big toenail. Pulling back

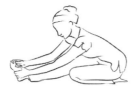

Figure Heart-7

on the toe, grab your foot with the left hand. Keep your chin tucked into the chest, spine straight, and eyes fixed on the big toe (Figure Heart-7). Inhale deeply. Exhale and hold the breath out for eight seconds, keeping Mūlbandh and Diaphragm Lock (page 94) tightly pulled. Inhale. Continue for three minutes. Relax on your back for five minutes.

Note: The Maha Mudra offers us a unique opportunity to be within. I find that holding the breath out in the manner described above works powerfully to shift the more etheric energies or spaces in the body where we tend to hold things.

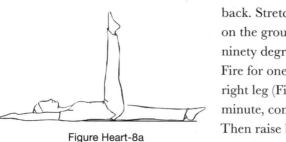

Figure Heart-8a

8. **Alternate Leg Lifts.** Lie on your back. Stretch your arms overhead on the ground. Raise the left leg ninety degrees and begin Breath of Fire for one minute. Switch to the right leg (Figure Heart-8a) for one minute, continuing Breath of Fire. Then raise both legs twelve inches only (Figure Heart-8b) and keep up the Breath of Fire for one more minute. Relax for two minutes.

Figure Heart-8b

9. **Shoulder Stand.** Slowly come into Shoulder Stand by raising the legs straight up toward the ceiling. Support the spine perpendicular to the ground with the hands, letting most of the weight rest on the elbows (Figure Heart-9). Spread your legs wide and begin Breath of Fire for three minutes. Relax on your back for three minutes.

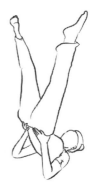

Figure Heart-9

10. **Alternate Head and Leg Lifts.** Lie on your back. Inhale and lift both legs six inches. Keep your arms straight up from the shoulders with palms facing in (Figure Heart-10a). On the exhale, lower both legs down and bring your head up, pressing the chin on your chest (Figure Heart-10b). Continue three minutes with long, deep breathing. Relax on your back for two minutes.

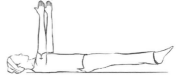

Figure Heart-10a

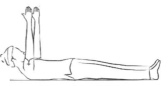

Figure Heart-10b

11. **Neck Rolls.** Sit in Easy Pose and hold opposite elbows across your chest. Roll your head in a slow figure eight for thirty seconds in one direction, then thirty seconds in the other direction (Figure Heart-11a). Then inhale deeply and bend forward to the ground (Figure Heart-11b). Exhale and rise up as fast as possible. Rise up and down ten times.

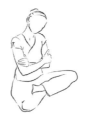

Figure Heart-11a

Figure Heart-11b

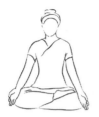

Figure Heart-12

12. Meditation. Sit in Easy Pose (Figure Heart-12) and chant "God and Me, Me and God, Are One." I recommend five to eleven minutes.

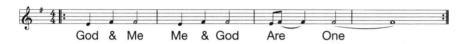

God & Me   Me & God   Are   One

Musical Notation for God and Me Meditation

Note: After practicing this Kriya, I recommend that you enjoy deep relaxation for five to eleven minutes on your back. After this, practice the Coming Out of Relaxation Exercises as described in chapter 6 (page 92).

PITUITARY GLAND SERIES

1. **Lunge Stretch.** Bend your right knee while keeping your right foot flat on the floor. Extend the left leg straight back and place your hands on the floor for balance (Figure Pituitary-1). Arch your head back and hold the position, breathing slowly and deeply for one minute. Keep the same posture and do Breath of Fire (page 94) for two minutes. Focus on your breathing for this exercise—it's the most difficult exercise in the set!

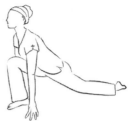

Figure Pituitary-1

2. **Lunge Stretch Rest.** From position 1, bring your right knee down to the floor and bend your torso to rest over the thigh. Place your forehead on the floor, stretch your left leg all the way back, and rest arms by the sides, palms up (Figure Pituitary-2). Breathe slowly and deeply for three minutes.

Figure Pituitary-2

3. Repeat exercises 1 and 2 with the opposite leg (Figure Pituitary-3).

Opposite of Exercise 2
Figure Pituitary-3

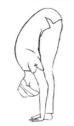

Figure Pituitary-4

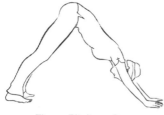

Figure Pituitary-5

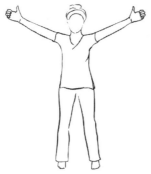

Figure Pituitary-6

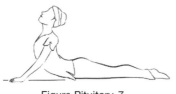

Figure Pituitary-7

4. **Front Bend.** Stand up with your feet hip-width apart. Bend over and touch your fingertips or palms on the floor (Figure Pituitary-4). Do long, deep breathing for three minutes.

5. **Ego Eradicator.** Stand up again and stretch your arms overhead at a thirty-degree angle, thumbs pointing up, fingers on palms (Figure Pituitary-5). Keep your elbows straight as you breathe long and deep for three minutes.

6. **Triangle Pose.** Rise onto your hands and knees and push up into Triangle Pose. Press your heels toward the floor while relaxing your head and neck (Figure Pituitary-6). Hold for up to three minutes.

7. **Cobra Pose.** Relax on your stomach for one minute. Then bring your heels together, palms flat on the floor under the shoulders. Push up into Cobra Pose (Figure Pituitary-7). Stretch your head and neck back and begin long, deep breathing for one minute. Then turn your head

from side to side, inhaling to the left, exhaling to the right. Continue for two minutes. Inhale, exhale, and pull Root Lock, or Mūlbandh (page 94), three times.

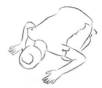

Figure Pituitary-8a

8. Sit on your heels and spread your knees far apart. Bring your forehead to the floor with palms flat on the ground in front of the knees (Figure Pituitary-8a). Inhale and rise up on your knees, stretching arms up and out like a flower greeting the sun (Figure Pituitary-8b). Exhale and fold down, bringing the forehead to the floor. Continue for three minutes.

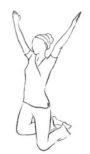

Figure Pituitary-8b

9. **Yoga Mudra.** Sit on your heels again with knees together and fingers interlaced at the base of the spine. Bring your forehead to the ground and lift arms up straight as far as possible (Figure Pituitary-9) and hold this position for three minutes with long, deep breathing.

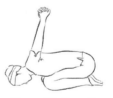

Figure Pituitary-9

Note: After this Kriya, I recommend that you enjoy deep relaxation for five to eleven minutes on your back. Afterward, practice the Coming Out of Relaxation Exercises as described in chapter 6 (page 92).

STRESS SET FOR ADRENALS AND KIDNEYS

Note: Practice the exercises in this set with very little rest between them.

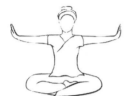

Figure Adrenals-1a

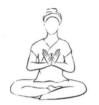

Figure Adrenals-1b

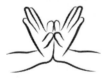

Figure Adrenals-1c

1. **Lotus Mudra.** In Easy Pose (page 98), rub your palms together. Inhale and stretch arms out to the sides, parallel to the ground, with palms facing out (Figure Adrenals-1a). Exhale and bring hands together in Lotus Mudra: base of palms together, thumbs and pinkie fingers touching, and the remaining fingers stretched open (Figure Adrenals-1b). Repeat for one to three minutes. To end, inhale with hands in Lotus Mudra (Figure Adrenals-1c).

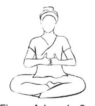

Figure Adrenals-2a

Figure Adrenals-2b

2. Interlace pinkies in front of the Heart Center, curling the other fingers into pads, thumbs sticking up. Lower your hands to the solar plexus (make sure your hands stay here and don't drift up) (Figure Adrenals-2a). Pull on the pinkies (Figure Adrenals-2b) and do Breath of Fire (page 94) from below the navel. Feel a pull across the back. Do this for one to three minutes.

3. **Cannon Breath.** Remain still in Easy Pose with straight spine. Relax your hands and begin Cannon Breath: Breath of Fire through a firm O-shaped mouth without allowing the cheeks to move (Figure Adrenals-3). Continue for one to three minutes and end by inhaling and concentrating on the spine.

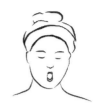

Figure Adrenals-3

4. In Easy Pose, place your left hand on your back at the bottom rib with your palm facing out. Extend your right arm straight out in front of you (Figure Adrenals-4a), flexing the wrist to create a sixty-degree angle in the hand (Figure Adrenals-4b). Keeping your spine straight, stretch from the shoulder. With eyes wide open, chant "har" powerfully from the navel. Do this for one to three minutes.

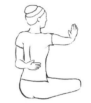

Figure Adrenals-4a

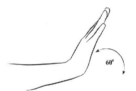

Figure Adrenals-4b

5. **Body Drops.** Come into Lotus Pose with the following steps. Sit with the legs stretched out in front of you. Bend the right leg at the knee toward you and put the right foot on the left thigh, then bend the left leg at the knee and place the left foot on top of the right thigh (Figure Adrenals-5a). You are welcome to reverse the sequence if you would like. If Lotus Pose is not possible for

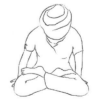

Figure Adrenals-5a

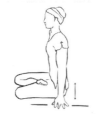

Figure Adrenals-5b

you, you can sit in Easy Pose. Place your hands on the ground by the sides of your body. Do Body Drops (Figure Adrenals-5b), inhaling as you push yourself up off the ground and exhaling as you drop down, continuing for one to three minutes. While doing this exercise, apply Neck Lock (page 94) and keep your spine erect. To protect your tongue, gently press your molars together.

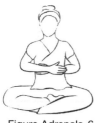

Figure Adrenals-6

6. In Easy Pose, place your hands in front of your solar plexus, left hand facing body, right hand pressing left wrist with the base of the palm (Figure Adrenals-6). With your head in Neck Lock, look down with powerful, long, deep breathing. Do this for one to three minutes.

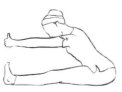

Figure Adrenals-7a

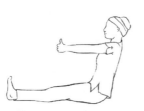

Figure Adrenals-7b

7. **Front Stretch with Spine Straight.** Sit with legs stretched out in front, arms out parallel to the ground, hands in fists, thumbs pointing up. Inhale, stretching forward (Figure Adrenals-7a); exhale, leaning back with powerful breath (Figure Adrenals-7b). Keep arms parallel to the ground on the inhale and the exhale. Continue for one to three minutes.

8. **Pelvic Lift.** Lying on your back, bend your knees and bring the soles of your feet flat onto the ground, heels at your buttocks. Grab your ankles. Inhale, lift the pelvis up (Figure Adrenals-8), and exhale down. Do this for one to three minutes.

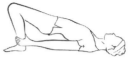

Figure Adrenals-8

9. **Modified Cat-Cow.** In cow position, exhale as you bring your left knee to the forehead (Figure Adrenals-9a). Inhale as you stretch your leg out and up in back (Figure Adrenals-9b). Do not overextend. Do this for one to three minutes, then switch to the right leg and repeat for another one to three minutes.

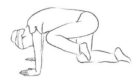

Figure Adrenals-9a

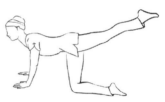

Figure Adrenals-9b

10. Sitting on your heels, bring forearms to the ground in front of your knees, palms together, thumbs pointing up (Figure Adrenals-10a). Inhale as you stretch over the palms (Figure Adrenals-10b), and exhale back. Keep your chin up to create pressure at the lower back. Continue for one to three minutes.

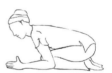

Figure Adrenals-10a

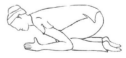

Figure Adrenals-10b

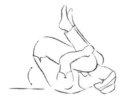

Figure Adrenals-11

11. **Back Rolls.** Lie on your back. Bring your knees to your chest, nose between knees. Breathe normally and roll back and forth on the spine for one to three minutes. (Figure Adrenals-11)

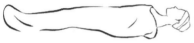

Figure Adrenals-12

12. **Totally Relax.** Enjoy Corpse Pose (Figure Adrenals-12) for one full hour, then drink a glass of water.

Note: I have practiced this set with notable results with only an eleven-minute relaxation on the back. As with other sets, practice the Coming Out of Relaxation Exercises as described in chapter 6 (page 92).

YOGA FOR MENSTRUAL HEALTH AND RELIEF

The following exercises can be done on a daily basis to support your menstrual health.[2]

1. **Tiger Stretch.** Sit on your right heel, left leg extended straight behind you. Stretch up with your forehead toward the sky. With your forearms at your ribs, bend your arms so the hands are at shoulder height, palms facing up (Figure Health-1). Hold the posture for up to five minutes with long, deep breathing. Repeat the exercise with the right leg back.

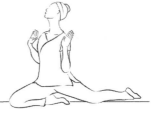

Figure Health-1

2. **Half Wheel Pose.** Lie down on your back and bring your heels to your buttocks with the feet flat on the floor. Grab your ankles, tighten the buttock muscles, and raise your torso up to the sky (Figure Health-2). Hold with long, deep breathing for up to three minutes. Gently come down and relax on your back. For an additional workout, you can inhale up and exhale down twenty-six times. I do not recommend doing this pose during the heavy flow of your cycle, as the uterus is inverted.

Figure Health-2

The following exercises can help relieve menstrual cramping. It is recommended to use full and relaxing breaths during the exercises and to take time to relax for three minutes or more after each one. You can do each exercise alone or as a set. Please evaluate each exercise and make sure that it feels good to your body before proceeding.

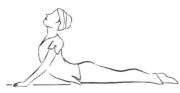

Figure Relief-1

1. **Cobra Pose.** Lie on your stomach with palms flat on the floor under your shoulders. Keep your heels together with the soles of the feet facing up. Press the hips into the ground and tighten the buttock muscles to inhale into Cobra Pose (Figure Relief-1). Lift the chest, allow the neck to lengthen, follow the curve of the upper back, and focus your eyes toward the sky with long, deep breathing for one minute.

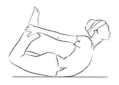

Figure Relief-2

2. **Bow Pose.** Lie on your stomach and bend your knees to grasp your ankles. Sink your hips into the floor, tighten your buttock muscles, and raise the thighs and head up off the floor (Figure Relief-2). Hold with long, deep breathing for two to three minutes.

3. **Bow Pose Variation.** If you can do Bow Pose easily for at least one minute, you may try this variation; otherwise please do not proceed. Bring yourself up into Bow Pose and rock back and forth on your stomach 108 times counting aloud. Enjoy a good sweat!

4. **Beginner's Locust Pose.** Lie on your belly with your hands in fists under your hips, just above the groin. With your chin on the floor and shoulders relaxed, bring your heels together, straighten your legs, and then raise your legs off the floor (Figure Relief-4). Hold with long, deep breathing for one to two minutes.

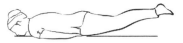

Figure Relief-4

5. **Leg Lift.** Lie on your back with the heels together and raise your legs up to a forty-five-degree angle from the floor (Figure Relief-5). Do your best to keep your legs straight and hold for up to three minutes with long, deep breathing. Relax in Corpse Pose with long, deep breathing.

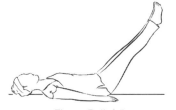

Figure Relief-5

~ *Appendix C* ~

AQUARIAN SĀDHANĀ MANTRAS

THE ĀDĪ SHAKTĪ MANTRA:
LONG EK ONG KĀR (Seven Minutes)

ek ong kār, sat nām sirī, wāhegurū.

*The Creator and all Creation are one, this is our true identity,
the ecstasy of wisdom is great beyond words.*

WĀH YANTĪ (Seven Minutes)

wāh yantī, kar yantī, jag dut patī, ādak it wāhā,
brahmāday trayshā gurū, it wāhegurū.

*Great Macroself, Creative Self.
All that is creative through time, all that is the Great One.
Three aspects of God: Brahma (Generator), Vishnu (Organizer),
Shiva (Deliverer) That is Wāhegurū.*

THE MŪL MANTRA (Seven Minutes)

ek ong kār, satinām, karatā purakh,
nirbha-u, nirvair, akāl mūrat, ajūnī, saibhang,
gur prasād, jap!
ād sach, jugād sach, hai bhī sach, nānak hosī bhī sach.

*God is One, Truth is God's Name, God is the Doer, without fear or vengeance,
Undying Form, Unborn, Self-illumined, Gurū's gift, repeat! True in the
beginning, true through the ages, true even now, oh Nānak, God is forever true.*

Sat Sirī Sirī Akāl (Seven Minutes)

sat sirī, sirī akāl, sirī akāl, mahā akāl,
mahā akāl, satinām, akāl mūrat, wāhegurū.

True and Great One, Great Undying One, Great Undying One, Exalted One, Undying One, Exalted One, Undying One, Truth is God's Name, Undying Form, great is the experience of Gurū; that One who brings us from darkness (gu) to light (rū).

Rakhay Rakhaṇahār (Seven Minutes)

rakhay rakhaṇahār āp ubāri-an, gur kī pairī pā-i kāj savāri-an,
ho-ā āp da-i-āl manah(u) na visāri-an, sādh janā kai sang bhavajal tāri-an,
sākat nindak dushṭ khin mā-he bidāri-an,
tis sāhib kī ṭayk nānak manai mā-he,
jis simarat sukh ho-i sagalay dūkh jā-he.

The Great Protector, the One who protects, that One who exists within us of Himself or Herself lifts us up. That One gave us the Lotus Feet of the Gurū on our foreheads and so all of our affairs and work are taken care of. God is merciful, kind, and compassionate so that we do not forget God in our mind. In the company of the Holy, we are carried across the challenges, calamities, and scandals of the world. Attachment to the world and slanderous enemies are destroyed. That great Lord is my anchor. Nānak, keep firm in your mind and cultivate the vibration of peace by meditating and repeating God's Name, and all happiness comes while sorrows and pain go away.

Wāhegurū Wāhe Jī-o (Twenty-Two Minutes)

wāhegurū, wāhegurū, wāhegurū, wāhe jī-o.

Ecstatic (Wāh!) is the experience of the Gurū, that One who brings us from darkness (gu) to light (rū). Ecstatic (Wāh!) is the experience of the Jī-o, the soul within that connects with the Divine Cosmic Soul of the One.

Gurū Rām Dās Chant (Five Minutes)

gurū gurū wāhegurū, gurū rām dās gurū.

This is in praise of the consciousness of Gurū Rām Dās, invoking his spiritual light, guidance, and protective grace. We are filled with humility.

~ *Appendix D* ~

ARDĀS — PRAYER

The traditional Sikh standing prayer, called Ardās, which is done in the fifth stage of the Aquarian Sādhanā, has an invocation that calls forth the energy of all eleven Sikh Gurūs to your aid, followed by a number of prayers and then a closing blessing.[1] The Ardās is recited by one person who comes forward and represents in consciousness and intention the prayers of all who are present.

In the "Open Prayer" section you can include prayers for people who need healing, recent births, or deaths. If someone has died, the community can chant the Mantra "Akāl!" (undying One) three times together, to help the soul merge with the Infinite.

The term *Khālsā* refers to those living in purity of conciousness.

Please rise to do your Ardās. If you are in a Gurdwārā, one would face the Sirī Gurū Granth Sāhib. If you are not in a Gurdwārā, I suggest facing toward your altar or that which you hold sacred. Hands are in prayer pose while you recite the following. When the Gurmukhī or transliteration is written, I suggest reciting these words as such to receive the blessings of the Naad.

ਅਰਦਾਸ

ARDĀS

Divine Prayer

ੴ ਸਿਰੀ ਵਾਹਿਗੁਰੂ ਜੀ ਕੀ ਫ਼ਤਹਿ !

ek ong kār sirī wāhegurū jī kī fateh!

There is One God and victory be to God!

ਸ੍ਰੀ ਭਗਉਤੀ ਜੀ ਸਹਾਇ ॥ ਵਾਰ ਸ੍ਰੀ ਭਗਉਤੀ ਜੀ ਕੀ ॥ ਪਾਤਸਾਹੀ ੧੦ ॥

sirī bhaga-utī jī sahā-i. vār sirī bhaga-utī jī kī pātasāhī dasavī.

*Oh Ādī Shaktī, may you protect us everywhere. This is the ballad of the
Ādī Shaktī composed by the tenth Master, Gurū Gobind Singh.*

ਪ੍ਰਿਥਮ ਭਗੌਤੀ ਸਿਮਰਿ ਕੈ ਗੁਰ ਨਾਨਕ ਲਈਂ ਧਿਆਇ ॥

pritham bhagautī simar kai guru nānak la-ī(n) dhi-ā-i.

After worshipping the Ādī Shaktī, the primal power, meditate on Gurū Nānak,

ਫਿਰ ਅੰਗਦ ਗੁਰ ਤੇ ਅਮਰਦਾਸੁ ਰਾਮਦਾਸੈ ਹੋਈਂ ਸਹਾਇ ॥

phir angad gur tay amaradās rāmadāsai ho-ī(n) sahā-i.

*Then Gurū Angad, Gurū Amar Das, and Gurū Rām Dās,
may they grant us their protection.*

ਅਰਜਨ ਹਰਿਗੋਬਿੰਦ ਨੋ ਸਿਮਰੌ ਸ੍ਰੀ ਹਰਿਰਾਇ ॥

arajan harigobind no simarau sirī harirā-i.

Worship Gurū Arjan, Gurū Hargobind, and Gurū Har Rai,

ਸ੍ਰੀ ਹਰਿ ਕਿਸ਼ਨ ਧਿਆਈਐ ਜਿਸ ਡਿਠੇ ਸਭਿ ਦੁਖਿ ਜਾਇ ॥

sirī har krishan dhi-ā-ī-ai jis ḍiṭhay sabh dukh jā-i.

Meditate on Gurū Har Krishan, upon seeing whom all sufferings depart.

ਤੇਗ ਬਹਾਦਰ ਸਿਮਰਿਐ ਘਰ ਨਉ ਨਿਧਿ ਆਵੈ ਧਾਇ ॥

tayg bahādar simari-ai ghar na-u nidh āvai dhā-i.

Meditate on Gurū Tegh Bahādur,
by whose grace the nine treasures come running to you.

ਸਭ ਥਾਈਂ ਹੋਇ ਸਹਾਇ ॥ ੧॥

sabh thā-ī(n) ho-i sahā-i. || 1||

O, Divine Masters, may you protect us everywhere.(1)

ਦਸਵੇਂ ਪਾਤਿਸ਼ਾਹ ਸ੍ਰੀ ਗੁਰੂ ਗੋਬਿੰਦ ਸਿੰਘ ਸਾਹਿਬ ਜੀ ਸਭ ਥਾਈਂ ਹੋਇ ਸਹਾਇ ॥

dasavay(n) patishah sirī gurū gobind singh
sahib jī sabh thā-ī(n) ho-i sahā-i.

Great Guru Gobind Singh, the tenth Guru, may you protect us everywhere.

ਦਸਾਂ ਪਾਤਿਸ਼ਾਹੀਆ ਦੀ ਜੋਤਿ ਸ੍ਰੀ ਗੁਰੂ ਗ੍ਰੰਥ ਸਾਹਿਬ ਜੀ,

dasa(n) patishahi-ā dī jot sirī gurū granth sāhib jī,

The light of the ten Gurūs, the living Gurū, the Sirī Gurū Granth Sāhib,

ਦੇ ਪਾਠ ਦੀਦਾਰ ਦਾ ਧਿਆਨ ਧਰ ਕੇ,

day paṭh dīdār dā dhi-ān dhar kay,

Grant us the blessing of Thy sacred word and a sight of Thy sacred form,

PRAYER LEADER CALLS OUT:

ਖਾਲਸਾ ਜੀ ਬੋਲੋ ਜੀ ਸਤਿਨਾਮੁ !

khālsā jī bolo jī, satinām!

Oh pure ones speak, Truth is God's Name!

COMMUNITY RESPONDS:

ਸ੍ਰੀ ਵਾਹਿਗੁਰੂ !

sirī wāhegurū!

Great is the experience of God!

May we remember all those who gave their lives
so that we may live as Khālsā today.

PRAYER LEADER CALLS OUT: **khālsā jī bolo jī, satinām!**

COMMUNITY RESPONDS: **sirī wāhegurū!**

May we remember and send prayers of prosperity and protection
to all Gurdwārās, and all holy places of God's worship.

PRAYER LEADER CALLS OUT: **khālsā jī bolo jī, satinām!**

COMMUNITY RESPONDS: **sirī wāhegurū!**

Let the whole Khālsā offer its prayer.
May the first prayer of the Khālsā be:

EVERYONE CHANTS: **wāhegurū, wāhegurū, wāhegurū.**

As we think of You, so may we be blessed. May Thy Grace and protection extend to all bodies of the Khālsā wherever we may be. May Thy Glory be fulfilled and Thy Will prevail. May we receive victory from the sword of righteousness and the charity of our brotherhood and sisterhood. May all of our work, businesses, schools, and efforts be divinely guided toward success, and may they be an offering to Thy Lotus Feet.

PRAYER LEADER CALLS OUT: **khālsā jī bolo jī, satinām!**

COMMUNITY RESPONDS: **sirī wāhegurū!**

Oh Lord, please give us the gift of discipline, and the blessing of your Name. May we have faith and confidence in Thee, and the ability to read and understand Thy sweet word. May we have a sight of and dip in the nectar tank of the Golden Temple. May the energy of the Golden Temple reside in our hearts. Bless us as people of conciousness with unity, love, and strength. May we live for each other. Please bless this earth with peace, bless this earth with peace, bless this earth with peace.

By your Grace, we have practiced this Aquarian Sādhanā. May our Sādhanā grow stronger every day. As we take this Hukam, may it penetrate our hearts and serve to draw our souls closer to you. Save us, oh Lord, from the five obtacles of lust, anger, greed, pride, and attachment. May we be attached only to Thy Lotus Feet. By Thy Grace, we have spent this night peacefully. May your Grace extend to the labors of this day that we may live in Thy Will.

Honor of the honorless, home of the homeless, strength of the weak, and hope of the hopeless. Oh True Gurū, shelter of the poor, we stand before Thee and offer our prayer.

Thank you for the teachings of the Siri Singh Sahib, Yogi Bhajan. May the legacy of these teachings stand strong and pure, and serve all of humanity with Thy blessings and love.

OPEN PRAYERS:

Note: You can offer prayers for healing by chanting "Akāl" three times for those who have recently passed, marriage blessings, or other pertinent prayers for you or your community. If Gur Prasād and Langar are available, you can do the following section.

GUR PRASĀD AND LANGAR BLESSING:

Please bless this Gur Prasād and Langar which have been lovingly placed before Thee. May its sweetness remind us of the sweetness of your Name, and the strength of the steel which cuts it remind us of the power of your Name to cut through all challenges.

Note: A community member would mark the blessing at this time by cutting through each with a Kirpān, or sacred sword, in a criss-cross pattern.

Please forgive us our errors and ommisions, and guide us in Thy way. May we be in the company of people of love so that we may remember Thy Name in their presence.

ਨਾਨਕੁ ਨਾਮ ਚੜ੍ਹਦੀ ਕਲਾ, ਤੇਰੇ ਭਾਣੇ ਸਰਬੱਤ ਦਾ ਭਲਾ ॥

nānak nām charadī kalā, tayray bhāṉay sarabat dā bhalā.

Through Nānak may Thy Name forever increase and the spirit be exalted, and may all people prosper by Thy Grace.

BOW DOWN WITH THE FOREHEAD TO THE FLOOR TO GIVE THE PRAYER TO GOD, AND RISE AGAIN TO SEND THE PRAYER OUT INTO THE COSMOS.

ਵਾਹਿਗੁਰੂ ਜੀ ਕਾ ਖਾਲਸਾ, ਵਾਹਿਗੁਰੂ ਜੀ ਕੀ ਫ਼ਤਹਿ !

Wāhegurū jī kā Khālsā, Wāhegurū jī kī Fateh!

The Khālsā belong to God, Victory belongs to God!

PRAYER LEADER CALLS:

ਬੋਲੇ ਸੋ ਨਿਹਾਲ !

bolay so nihāl!

Speak with joy!

COMMUNITY RESPONDS:

ਸਤਿ ਸਿਰੀ ਅਕਾਲ !

sat sirī akāl!

Great and true is the Undying One!

BOW DOWN TO SEAL THE PRAYER.

RESOURCES

TO STUDY MORE IN DEPTH WITH ME

- Sign up for my newsletter at snatamkaur.com or at facebook/SnatamKaur to find out more about music, workshops, festivals, Naad Yoga courses, and more.

- Attend a workshop with me.

- Take a Naad Yoga course.

- Check out the different festivals where I teach (for example, Sat Nam Fest, Summer Solstice, or Winter Solstice).

- Attend a concert where I play with other musicians.

TO LEARN JAP JĪ

Meditation of the Soul: Jap Jī Daily Practice and Learning Tool: This is a set of two CDs and a book I created to help you learn or strengthen your Jap Jī practice. See spiritvoyage.com/meditationofthesoul for more information.

SĀDHANĀ AROUND THE WORLD

To experience a powerful community Sādhanā practice, attend one of these incredible events:

- **Summer and Winter Solstice Sādhanā Celebrations.** At these incredible events, we enjoy three days of White Tantric Yoga, an all-night sacred music experience, a Morning Sādhanā with two thousand yogīs for the summer gathering, and a yogic diet. After attending this event, I feel entirely cleansed and uplifted.

In winter we gather in Florida, and in summer we meet in the mountains of northern New Mexico. See 3HO.org for more information.

- **Sat Nam Fest.** Two of these Kundalini Yoga and music festivals take place every year: in the spring in Joshua Tree and in the fall in Massachusetts. Beautiful musicians and yoga teachers of my community gather and share sacred experiences and teachings of Kundalini Yoga, meditation, and chanting. You'll also find a wonderful children's program, as well. See satnamfest.com for more information.

- **European Yoga Festival.** This summer festival occurs in France where over two thousand people gather from various countries, practice three days of White Tantric Yoga, and enjoy classes with incredible teachers and musicians from all over the world. See 3HO-europe.org for more information.

OTHER COMMUNITY RESOURCES

- If you are just starting out, try to attend a weekly Kundalini Yoga class. To find a certified Kundalini Yoga teacher near you, look at IKYTA.org.

- To download music and DVDs from me or from other artists and teachers of the 3HO community, check out spiritvoyage.com. You can also use the link to find online global Sādhanās to attend from the comfort of your own home.

- To download other books, DVDs, and resources for Kundalini Yoga, or to find a course near you to become a certified Kundalini Yoga teacher, use kundaliniresearchinstitute.org.

- My favorite research website is the Yogi Bhajan Library of Teachings. It is the archival library of Yogi Bhajan's published lectures and Kriya write-ups in searchable text, audio, and video formats. Find it at libraryofteachings.com.

- To learn about Sikh history or Yogi Bhajan's teachings on Sikh Dharma, to connect with the global Sikh community, or to download useful apps that aid in the practices of the Sikh way of life, check out sikhnet.com.

- To connect with the Sikh Dharma community, tap into educational resources both online and via courses, or order Sikh books and manuals, use sikhdharma.org.

- To attend a telecourse to help you learn about Sikh Dharma, try journeyintotheheartofsikhdharma.org.

RECOMMENDED READING

These are some of my favorite books on Kundalini Yoga:

- Bhajan, Yogi. *The Master's Touch.* Santa Cruz, NM: Kundalini Research Institute, 1997.

- Bhajan, Yogi, and Singh Khalsa, Gurucharan. *The Mind: Its Projections and Multiple Facets.* Santa Cruz, NM: Kundalini Research Institute, 1998.

- Khalsa, Guru Meher. *Senses of the Soul: Emotional Therapy for Strength, Healing, and Guidance.* Santa Cruz, NM: Kundalini Research Institute, 2013.

- Khalsa, Shakti Parwha Kaur. *Kundalini Yoga: The Flow of Eternal Power.* New York: Perigee Books, 1998.

- Khalsa, Jot Singh. *The Essential Element: How to Get the Most out of Yogi Bhajan's Core Teaching—Morning Sadhana, and Why You Won't Want to Miss It.* Millis, MA: Jot Singh Khalsa, 2014.

The following books are specifically for women:

- Bhajan, Yogi. *I Am a Woman.* Santa Cruz, NM: Kundalini Research Institute, 2009.

- Khalsa, Sangeet Kaur. *Womanheart: Healing Our Relationships, Loving Ourselves.* Phoenix, AZ: Womanheart Publishing, 2002.

- Khalsa, Sat Purkh Kaur. *Everyday Grace: The Art of Being a Woman.* Santa Cruz, NM: Kundalini Research Institute, 2010.

- Seibel, Machelle M., and Khalsa, Hari Kaur. *A Woman's Book of Yoga.* New York: Penguin Putnam, 2002.

Find out more about women's camp at 3HO.org and learn more about conscious pregnancy at Kundaliniwomen.org or goldenbridgeyoga.com.

For courses, books, and information on Ayurveda, explore Ayurveda.com, kripalu.org, or jaidevsingh.com.

To find out more about sacred sex and conception, read:

- Khalsa, Sat Kaur. *Sacred Sexual Bliss: A Technology for Ecstasy.* Santa Cruz, NM: Yogi Ji Press, 2000.

- Khalsa, Guru Terath Kaur. *The Art of Making Sex Sacred: Techniques for Intimate Relationships.* Santa Cruz NM: Yogi Ji Press, 1998.

CHILDREN'S RESOURCES

- **Khalsa Youth Camp.** Kids between five and twelve learn yoga, meditation, martial arts, and music in such a way that supports the radiance of spirit and self-esteem. I serve as the Sikh Dharma teacher, focusing on the universal aspects of spirituality from the Sikh tradition through music and stories. See 3HO.org for more information.

- **Miri Piri Academy.** This boarding school founded by Yogi Bhajan serves kids age eight through high school in Amritsar, India. This academy gives children a strong spiritual foundation through the practice of yoga, meditation, sacred music, martial arts, and service. It also entails a strong academic program. Children from all over the world attend and create lifelong friendships. Check out miripiriacademy.org.

- **Children's Music and DVDs from Snatam Kaur.** *Shanti the Yogi* is a yoga class with me and a group of children that includes illustrations, music, and an imaginative story. *Feeling Good Today,* my first CD for children, includes upbeat Mantras and positive affirmations from Yogi Bhajan. *Sat Nam! Songs from Khalsa Youth Camp* contains songs that highlight self-esteem and joy.

RECORDINGS OF STANZAS OF JAP JĪ FROM SNATAM KAUR

- From the album *Ras:* "So Mai Visar Na Jaa-ee"

- From *Anand:* "Mul Mantra"

- From *Shanti:* "Ek Ong Kaar," "Dayndaa Day—Infinity," "Aakhan Jor—Acceptance," "Suni-ai—Listening Meditation," and "Sun-ai—Listening Celebration"

MUSIC AND DVDS FROM SNATAM KAUR

For the many music albums and yoga DVDs that I have had the blessing to create, please visit snatamkaur.com.

NOTES

Introduction

1. The Teachings of Yogi Bhajan, October 4, 1987.

Chapter One: The Gift of Practice

1. *Amrit Kīrtan* (Amritsar, India: Khalsa Brothers, 1981), 208.
2. Sant Singh Khalsa, *Sundar Gutkaa* (Tucson: Handmade Books, 2000), 31.
3. Yogi Bhajan and Gurucharan Singh Khalsa, *The Mind: Its Projections and Multiple Facets* (Santa Cruz, NM: Kundalini Research Institute, 1998), 75.
4. Snatam Kaur, *Feeling Good Today!* (Spirit Voyage, 2009) compact disc. Lyrics by Yogi Bhajan.
5. Yogi Bhajan, *The Aquarian Teacher* (Santa Cruz, NM: Kundalini Research Institute, 2005), 4–8.
6. Bhajan, *The Aquarian Teacher*, 6.

Chapter Two: Sacred Sound As Teacher

1. Khalsa, *Sundar Gutkaa*, 24.
2. Bhajan, *The Aquarian Teacher*, chapter 7.
3. Max Arthur MacAuliffe, *The Sikh Religion* (Delhi, India: Low Price Publications, 1996).
4. Bhajan, *The Aquarian Teacher*, 73–77.

Chapter Three: A Journey into Kundalini

1. *Amrit Kīrtan*, 738.
2. Sant Singh Khalsa, trans., *Siri Guru Granth Sahib Ji* (Española, NM: Sikhnet, 2014), 1, 399.
3. Bhajan, *The Aquarian Teacher*, 184–195.
4. Bhajan, *The Aquarian Teacher*, 174.

5. Bhajan, *The Aquarian Teacher,* 180, 324.

6. Bhajan, *The Aquarian Teacher,* 70–77.

7. Bhajan, *The Aquarian Teacher,* 73–77.

8. Yogi Bhajan, *Kundalini Yoga Sadhana Guidelines,* 2nd ed. (Santa Cruz, NM: Kundalini Research Institute, 2007), 16.

9. Bhajan, *The Aquarian Teacher,* 201–204.

10. MacAuliffe, *The Sikh Religion.*

11. Bhajan, *The Aquarian Teacher,* 203.

12. Bhajan, *Kundalini Yoga Sadhana Guidelines,* 16.

Chapter Four: Altar of the Self
Stage One: Preparing for the Aquarian Sādhanā

1. Khalsa, *Siri Guru Granth Sahib Ji,* 1158.

2. Khalsa, *Sundar Gutkaa,* 4.

3. Shakti Parwha Kaur Khalsa, *Kundalini Yoga: The Flow of Eternal Power* (New York: Perigee Books, 1998), 122.

4. Benjamin Franklin, *Poor Richard's Almanack* (Published by Benjamin Franklin, 1735).

5. Bhajan, *The Aquarian Teacher,* 247.

6. Bhajan, *The Aquarian Teacher,* 151,178, 249.

7. Khalsa, *Kundalini Yoga: The Flow of Eternal Power,* 119–120. Hari Simran Singh, *The Hue-man* (Golden Dragon Productions, 2012), 26, 46, 83.

8. Bhajan, *The Aquarian Teacher,* 138.

9. Dr. Hari Simran Singh Khalsa, email to author, June 5, 2015.

10. Bhajan, *The Aquarian Teacher,* 151,178, 249.

Chapter Five: Meditation of the Soul
Stage Two: Jap Jī

1. Khalsa, *Siri Guru Granth Sahib Ji,* 318.

2. MacAuliffe, *The Sikh Religion.*

3. Guru Kirn Kaur Khalsa, *Living with the Guru* (New Delhi, India: Wisdom Tree, 2006).

4. The Teachings of Yogi Bhajan, July 19, 1989.

5. Bhajan, *The Aquarian Teacher,* 79–80.

6. The Teachings of Yogi Bhajan, April 16, 1985.

7. Khalsa, *Sundar Gutkaa*, 31.

8. Machelle M. Seibel and Hari Kaur Khalsa, *A Woman's Book of Yoga* (New York: Penguin Putnam, 2002), 57.

9. The Teachings of Yogi Bhajan, April 16, 1985.

10. Ek Ong Kaar Kaur Khalsa, *Japji Sāhib for Sadhana*, May 10, 2014.

Chapter Six: Bliss in the Body
Stage Three: Kundalini Yoga

1. Khalsa, *Siri Guru Granth Sahib Ji*, 92.

2. Yogi Bhajan, *The Aquarian Teacher Level One Instructor Manual* (Santa Cruz, NM: Kundalini Research Institute, 2003), 13.

3. Hari Kirin Kaur Khalsa, email to author, July 23, 2015.

4. Bhajan, *The Aquarian Teacher*, 54.

5. Harijot Kaur, ed., *Self-Experience* (Santa Cruz, NM: Kundalini Research Institute, 2000).

6. Bhajan, *The Aquarian Teacher*, Level One Instructor Manual, 18.

7. Bhajan, *The Aquarian Teacher*, 118.

8. Gurucharan Singh Khalsa, *The 21 Stages of Meditation* (Santa Cruz, NM: Kundalini Research Institute, 2012).

9. Khalsa, *The 21 Stages of Meditation*.

Chapter Seven: Chanting as the Sun Rises
Stage Four: Aquarian Sādhanā Mantras

1. Khalsa, *Siri Guru Granth Sahib Ji*, 1316.

2. The Teachings of Yogi Bhajan, July 20, 1989.

3. C. A. Shackle, *A Gurū Nānak Glossary* (Vancouver, Canada: University of British Columbia Press, 1981).

4. Khalsa, *The 21 Stages of Meditation*.

5. Bhajan, *The Aquarian Teacher*, 215.

6. Shackle, *A Gurū Nānak Glossary*.

7. The Teachings of Yogi Bhajan, June 29, 1995.

8. Shackle, *A Gurū Nānak Glossary*.

9. Yogi Bhajan, *The Master's Touch* (Santa Cruz, NM: Kundalini Research Institute, 1997), 97.

10. Shackle, *A Gurū Nānak Glossary.*
11. Bhajan, *The Master's Touch,* 135.
12. Swami Chidanand Saraswati, *Drops of Nectar* (New Delhi, India: Wisdom Tree, 2006), 204.
13. Bhajan and Khalsa, *The Mind,* 155.
14. Shackle, *A Gurū Nānak Glossary.*
15. Shackle, *A Gurū Nānak Glossary.*
16. Bhajan, *The Aquarian Teacher,* 326.
17. Nirvair Singh Khalsa, email to author, June 6, 2014.
18. *Amrit Kīrtan,* 281.
19. The Teachings of Yogi Bhajan, June 6, 1996.
20. Shackle, *A Gurū Nānak Glossary.*

Chapter Eight: Surrender, Bow, and Receive
Stage Five: Gateway to Divinity

1. Khalsa, *Sundar Gutkaa,* 160.
2. Khalsa, *Sundar Gutkaa,* 4.
3. Mike Heron, "Long Time Sun" (Warner-Tamerlane, 2004). Used by permission of Alfred Music.

Chapter Nine: Presence of Self

1. Khalsa, *Siri Guru Granth Sahib Ji,* 968.
2. Bhajan, *The Aquarian Teacher,* 150.
3. Bhajan, *The Aquarian Teacher,* 144–146.

Chapter Ten: Blessings for Family and Community

1. Khalsa, *Siri Guru Granth Sahib Ji,* 278.
2. H. H. Pujya Swami Chidanand Saraswatiji, 2013 Calendar, Parmarth Niketan Ashram, parmarth.com.
3. Tarn Taran Kaur Khalsa, *Conscious Pregnancy: The Gift of Giving Life* (Española, NM: Kundalini Women, 2008).
4. Sikhnet Stories, sikhnet.com.
5. Bhajan, *The Master's Touch,* 202.
6. Bhajan, *The Aquarian Teacher,* 146.

Epilogue

1. Yogi Bhajan, *Japji Sahib-Lecture,* Part 1, The Teachings of Yogi Bhajan, July 16–18, 2003, sikhnet.com/video/japji-sahib-lecture-yogi-bhajan-part-1.

Appendix A: Jap Jī Sāhib

1. Khalsa, *Sundar Gutkaa,* 1–32.

Appendix B: Kundalini Yoga Sets

1. Bhajan, *The Aquarian Teacher Level One Instructor Manual,* 10–13, 17, 18, 24, 25, 36–39, 43, 44, 47.
2. Seibel and Khalsa, *A Woman's Book of Yoga,* 76–82.

Appendix D: Ardās—Prayer

1. Sources of translation: Shackle, *A Gurū Nānak Glossary.* Khalsa, *Sundar Gutkaa,* 157. Premka Kaur, *Peace Lagoon* (Española, NM: Sikh Dharma International).

About the Author

Snatam Kaur is an American singer and peace activist raised in the Sikh and Kundalini Yoga tradition. She has an amazing ability to transform traditional Sikh chants of India into a contemporary sound that appeals to the modern ear and awakens an ancient yearning in the soul. For over thirty years, she studied with and grew up in the presence of her spiritual teacher, Yogi Bhajan, while he was in his physical form, learning the essence of Naad Yoga, a form of yoga focusing on sacred sound. At the core of this practice is an essential experience of peace and healing, which has helped her music to be accessible to people of all walks of life. She has taught and shared Naad Yoga and Kundalini Yoga and meditation through her recorded CDs, concerts, and workshops for the past fifteen years, as a part of her commitment to give people tools for a daily experience of inner peace.

ABOUT SPIRIT VOYAGE

Spirit Voyage is a sacred chant record lable, event producer, music distributor, and Kundalini Yoga lifestyle company. Spirit Voyage was born of the belief that the power of Kundalini Yoga and sacred music can transform the planet, one person at a time.

We believe in this music. We believe in this yoga.

We believe in the light of these teachers who spread beauty and grace with their voices, lifting us all to our highest selves.

We are a company created to serve.

For more information, please visit spiritvoyage.com or call us toll-free at 888.735.4800.

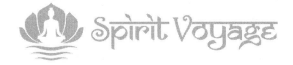

ABOUT SOUNDS TRUE

Sounds True is a multimedia publisher whose mission is to inspire and support personal transformation and spiritual awakening. Founded in 1985 and located in Boulder, Colorado, we work with many of the leading spiritual teachers, thinkers, healers, and visionary artists of our time. We strive with every title to preserve the essential "living wisdom" of the author or artist. It is our goal to create products that not only provide information to a reader or listener, but that also embody the quality of a wisdom transmission.

For those seeking genuine transformation, Sounds True is your trusted partner. At SoundsTrue.com you will find a wealth of free resources to support your journey, including exclusive weekly audio interviews, free downloads, interactive learning tools, and other special savings on all our titles.

To learn more, please visit SoundsTrue.com/freegifts or call us toll-free at 800.333.9185.

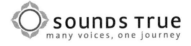